SCHERING

Contrast-Enhanced MRI of the Breast

Sylvia H. Heywang-Köbrunner

Dr. Sylvia H. Heywang-Köbrunner
Klinikum Großhadern
Radiologische Klinik
Marchioninistraße 15
D-8000 München 70

Published in the medico-scientific book series of Schering

The book shop edition is published by Karger Basel – München – Paris – London – New York – New Delhi – Bangkok – Singapore – Tokyo – Sydney

Where reference is made to the use of Schering products, the reader is advised to consult the latest scientific information issued by the company.

Publishers: HD Med. Information,
Sektion Medizinische Redaktion, Schering
Design: Werbestudio of Schering in collaboration with Urte von Bremen
Anatomical drawings: Darja Süßbier
Copyediting: Editorial Experts, Inc., Alexandria, VA, USA
Lithography: JUP Industrie- und Presseklischee, Berlin
Composition and print: Druckerei Hellmich KG, Berlin
Printed in Germany
© Copyright 1990 by Schering
ISBN 3-8055-5293-9

NIGEL McMILLAN

MRI DEPT.

W.I.G.

Contrast-Enhanced MRI of the Breast

Contents

Foreword

This book is the fruit of six years of work by Dr. Sylvia H. Heywang-Köbrunner on the use of magnetic resonance (MR) imaging to investigate the female breast. It is a tribute to Dr. Heywang's commitment to the task and a testimony to the extraordinary results that she has achieved, results that fully justify publication in book form.

Although MR imaging has not yet become a routine method of investigating the breast, Dr. Heywang makes it abundantly clear that this method, especially with the use of contrast media, is an almost ideal complementary procedure in cases in which neither mammography nor ultrasound yields an unequivocal result. In such cases patients need not be left in the dark. MR imaging may obviate the need for biopsy or at least ensure that it is performed in the right place and at the right time. In this situation, we have found MR imaging of the breast to be valuable and important in diagnosis and aftercare.

Dr. Heywang deserves credit for having developed this method of investigation from abstract idea to practical clinical application. I offer her my heartfelt congratulations on her accomplishment.

Professor Dr. Dr. Josef Lissner, Munich 1990

Preface

Since our first application of Gd-DTPA (gadolinium diethylene triamine pentaacetic acid) for magnetic resonance (MR) imaging of the female breast* in 1985, contrast-enhanced MRI has become a more and more interesting method of examination which promises to improve diagnostic accuracy in conjunction with other modalities. The increasing amount of attention the method has received suggested the need for an overview of current research.

This book addresses all those interested in further research and development in breast imaging and MRI and provides a survey of possibilities, limitations, and indications of this new method to gynecologists, surgeons, and radiologists.

The book is based mainly on research at the Klinikum Großhadern, University of Munich, but also includes and discusses current MRI research worldwide.

* Gd-DTPA is still under review. Gd-DTPA has not yet been approved for this indication.

Acknowledgements

For making this work possible at all and for his continuous support I am deeply grateful to Professor Dr. med. Dr. hc. J. Lissner, Head of Radiology, Klinikum Großhadern, University of Munich.

I also wish to express my profound thanks to Dr. H.-P. Niendorf and Dr. W. Clauß from Schering for their excellent and constant support in the development of the method and the book.

My sincere thanks also go to Siemens Corporation, especially the UB Medizinische Technik Erlangen and the Medizinische Technik München Region Süd, for their constantly available cooperation and expertise.

I am very thankful for the grants and the continuous support this project has received since 1985 from Deutsche Krebshilfe, Mildred-Scheel-Stiftung.

I acknowledge with deep appreciation the meticulous work of Prof. W. Permanetter (Department of Pathology, Klinikum Großhadern, Head: Prof. Dr. M. Eder), who not only contributed excellent histopathologic correlations and advice, but also helped us to interpret and understand MRI findings based on histopathologic changes.

My sincere thanks go to all of the clinicians and radiologists who supported this project, especially to Prof. Dr. W. Eiermann and Dr. K. Diergarten (Department of Gynecology, Klinikum Großhadern, Head: Prof. Dr. H. Hepp), who referred most of our patients, and who also offered the encouragement, scientific interest, and expertise that made the clinical correlations and patient surveys possible.

I thank all of my colleagues who supported this project, especially Dr. Th. Hilbertz and Dr. R. Beck, who spent many hours with me examining patients, evaluating studies, and improving the method.

A special note of gratitude must be accorded to Ms. A. Plesch and Ms. U. Ritter, who gathered the material and typed the manuscript.

Many thanks also go to our photographers, for their fast and excellent help in preparing the illustrative material.

Finally, I am very grateful to Ms. A. Schlemmer and Dr. K. Friebel of Schering, Medizinische Redaktion, for their excellent editing of the manuscript, to Editorial Experts, Inc., Karger publishers and Ms. U. von Bremen for their fast and professional work.

List of abbreviations

CHESS	chemical shift selection
3D	three dimensional
FA	flip angle
FI	fast imaging
FISP	fast imaging with steady state precession = a gradient echo fast imaging pulse sequence
FLASH	fast low angle shot = a gradient echo fast imaging pulse sequence
Gd-DTPA	gadolinium diethylene triamine pentaacetic acid
LCIS	lobular carcinoma in situ
MRI	magnetic resonance imaging
NU	normalized units, see page 31
PEACH	paramagnetic enhancement accentuated by chemical shift
RT	radiation therapy
SE	spin echo
S/N ratio	signal-to-noise ratio
STIR	short TI inversion recovery
T1	longitudinal relaxation time
T2	transverse relaxation time
TE	echo time
TI	inversion time
TR	repetition time

Introduction

Since its introduction* contrast-enhanced magnetic resonance imaging (MRI) of the breast has gained increased attention.

The different information it offers compared to the other imaging modalities is proving especially helpful in diagnostically difficult cases. Due to its own limitations (high costs, large number of slices per breast, limited specificity in cases with diffuse enhancement), it should not be used alone and will not replace mammography. As a supplementary tool, however, it has proven very effective and valuable, because it helps to increase both specificity and sensitivity.

For these reasons contrast-enhanced MRI will not be treated alone in this book, but in close connection with the other methods used in breast diagnostics.

The introductory sections (pages 11-19) give an overview of the present state of breast imaging. Weak points of conventional breast diagnostics are emphasized to attract attention to those areas where additional information is desirable. A short overview follows of the present state of plain MRI, which has not been as successful as initially hoped. Finally the principles and state of contrast-enhanced MRI are briefly described.

The second section (pages 20-45) treats the technique of contrast-enhanced MRI in general and our own standard examination, including some practical advice. Detailed information is given especially for those interested in the application of contrast-enhanced MRI.

The third section (pages 46–176) gives an overview of the MRI appearance of various lesions, followed by general criteria and simplified guidelines for MRI interpretation and its influence on further work-up. It first describes each entity's specific histopathologic features that influence MRI appearance. Possibilities and limitations of conventional imaging follow, and special problems in the differential diagnosis are reviewed. Finally the normal MRI appearance, including exceptions, are described and both differential diagnosis of the various appearances and the potential value of MRI in a multimodality approach are worked out.

* We developed this method and introduced it in 1985.

The fourth section (pages 177–230) first presents data concerning the accuracy of contrast-enhanced MRI of the breast. Then indications for a useful application of MRI in the clinical setting are proposed and discussed, followed by typical examples in the form of case reports.

The last section (pages 231-232) reminds us that MRI is still a matter of research. Thus, both desirable optimizations and future aspects are considered.

Conventional breast diagnostics: possibilities, limitations and questions regarding new modalities

Affecting 1 of 11 women, breast cancer has become the most important cause of death in women (10). Based on large studies (25, 29, 108, 109, 119) the importance of screening is more and more widely accepted. The major goals of breast diagnostics are early detection of malignancy and its differentiation from other breast disease.

So far, the following methods have been available:
For screening, a combined evaluation by mammography and clinical examination has proven most effective. For further differentiation of mammographic or clinical abnormalities, methods such as sonography or cytology have proven quite helpful (11, 12, 34, 37, 74, 86, 88). Thermography or transillumination are not generally accepted due to their high number of false positive and false negative calls (3, 31, 92, 120).

Since even the accepted methods are not infallible, knowledge of the limitations of each method is crucial.

Mammography provides a sensitivity of almost 100% in the fatty breast. Thus, in fatty areas malignancy can be excluded even in the presence of a palpable abnormality. Small irregular densities, which are excellently imaged in the fatty breast, may be the only sign of a small nonpalpable malignancy. The other strength of mammography is the excellent demonstration of microcalcifications, which are present in about 30-50% of early malignancies (77). In the dense (radiopaque) and very dense breast, however, the sensitivity of mammography significantly decreases (7, 62, 96). Whereas tumors with microcalcifications are still quite reliably identified, those without microcalcifications may be obscured by overlying breast tissue. Unless subtle architectural distortion, retraction, asymmetry, or some change with time attracts the mammographer's attention, tumors that exhibit the same radio-density as the surrounding dense breast tissue are invisible.

For this reason combined evaluation by mammography and clinical examination is essential, and as a rule malignancy cannot be excluded within mammographically dense areas if a palpable abnormality exists. This fact is also documented by the significant number of tumors that are detected by clinical abnormalities only (7, 65).

Even though some very small tumors may be detected by palpation or clinical examination alone, the majority of palpable lesions exceed 1 cm. This fact is not only due to the impossibility of feeling small lesions deep in a large breast. The distinction between individual normal and abnormal thickening or lumpiness may be quite difficult to make, depending as it does on the highly variable consistency of normal and abnormal tissue.

Ultrasound is most useful in distinguishing between solid mass and cyst and thus helps avoid unnecessary biopsies. Since mammographically dense tissue usually is quite echogenic and since most carcinomas are hypoechoic (with or without shadowing), ultrasound can also be used to confirm a palpable malignancy within mammographically dense tissue. However, since some malignancies – especially noninvasive and diffusely growing carcinomas – may not be visible sonographically, ultrasound cannot be used to exclude malignancy. Furthermore, its sensitivity decreases in the absence of a palpable abnormality and with smaller lesions (34, 74, 86).

Cytology is helpful in selected cases (37, 88). However, owing to its known lower accuracy rate, cytology is generally not accepted as substitute for histology. Especially if the findings are negative, one needs to bear in mind the possibility of sampling beside the lesion (which may happen especially with small lesions). In addition, fibrotic lesions (like scirrhous carcinomas or scarring) may not allow aspiration of sufficient material from the lesion even if the needle is placed exactly. Small-cell malignancies (like the lobular carcinoma) often cannot be differentiated from benign lesions by the cytologist because of their uniform appearance. Finally, indeterminate microcalcifications are frequently found beside a malignancy. Therefore, negative cytology is not as reliable as positive cytology. In spite of the latest exact stereotactic techniques, the value of cytology especially in nonpalpable lesions is still the object of significant controversy (9, 12, 27, 105, 122).

Depending on the diagnostic question and on the experience and equipment available for the different methods, the diagnostician finally has to choose the best individual combination of methods to use. In addition, comparison with previous studies (if available and of comparable quality) is usually quite helpful and is therefore always attempted. Knowing the advantages and limitations of the various methods makes an accurate diagnosis possible in the great majority of cases.

In a certain percentage of diagnostically difficult cases, however, an accurate diagnosis is almost impossible, even for the experienced diagnostician. Such problems include for example the following:

– Exclusion or demonstration of malignancy in mammographically dense tissue with uncertain palpable and/or sonographic findings.

– Differentiation of uncharacteristic mammographic densities, asymmetries, or microcalcifications.

– Differentiation of mammographic or palpable questionable abnormalities in patients with extensive scarring, with silicon implants, or after lumpectomy and radiation therapy.

– Distinction between chronic or acute mastitis and malignancy.

Concerning the further management of such cases, the following facts have to be considered:

Diagnostic biopsies of benign pathology should be kept as low as possible. This is desirable to avoid unnecessary fear and operations with possible complications and extensive scarring, which may complicate future diagnoses. Many biopsies with benign pathology also risk decreased confidence in the diagnostic capabilities and decreased patient compliance. However, precious time may elapse before change of a suspicious lesion is documented on follow-up examinations.

These considerations are even more important with the increased use of screening necessary for early detection, since we know that with decreasing size of the abnormality in question the specificity of all methods falls significantly. Depending on the "aggressiveness of screening for small lesions", biopsy rates ranging from 1:2 to 1:10 (corresponding to 1 cancer in 2 or 10 recommended biopsies respectively) have been reported for nonpalpable lesions detected by screening (1, 14, 26, 36, 77, 93, 112).

In summary, a number of excellent methods are already available for early detection and differentiation of breast carcinoma. Because of technical progress and increasing experience, smaller carcinomas can now be detected. Nevertheless, more information is still desirable to increase sensitivity in mammographically dense breasts and to improve specificity, especially for differentiation of small lesions. For this reason other methods, including MRI, are being investigated. Most progress has been achieved by contrast-enhanced MRI, which is more and more clinically accepted.

Plain MRI of the breast: principle and results

Initial reports raised the hope that an improved tissue characterization might become possible by evaluating the MRI properties of the different breast tissues (18, 23, 83, 104). These properties can be assessed in two different ways:

– By evaluation of the so-called tissue parameters T1, T2, and proton density.

– Directly by evaluation of the signal intensities the tissues assume on different pulse sequences.

Tissue differentiation based on tissue parameters calculated from in vivo MR imaging turned out to be more difficult than expected, and significant overlap was found between the values of benign and malignant lesions (2, 47, 95, 97, 124). Reasons for this insufficient distinction include technical problems (determination of T1 or T2 from a low number of measurements, influence of imaging gradients and slice profile on accuracy) and biological causes (motion artifacts and motion between the measurements, partial volume effect, multiexponential T1 or T2 decays, and possibly similar biochemical composition of benign and malignant tissues).

Even though pulse sequences for T1 and T2 determinations have been refined and accuracy has improved (30, 43, 87), a sufficient tissue differentiation has not been achieved by evaluating tissue parameters.

Evaluation of the change of tissue signal intensity with different pulse sequences in principle offers the same information as evaluation of tissue parameters, since the signal intensity is determined by T1, T2, and proton density of the tissue and by the imaging parameters of each pulse sequence. Nevertheless, such an evaluation so far appears more promising. The information provided by the direct image is easier to interpret and inaccuracies that may occur in the calculation of tissue parameters need not be considered.

Comparative histopathologic studies have shown a good correlation between the signal intensity of the tissue on T2-weighted SE sequences and its content of fibrosis, cells, or water. Fibrous tissue displays the lowest signal intensity on T2-weighted pulse sequences whereas high cell or water content correlates with intermediate to high signal intensities (24, 45, 47, 76, 95, 115, 124).

This MRI feature in fact has proven advantageous for the demonstration of the internal structure of some lesions (e. g., central fibrosis, central necrosis) and – more important – for the distinction between fibrous fibroadenomas with low signal intensity and the other well-circumscribed solid lesions (like some carcinomas, metastases, cystosarcomas, and myxoid and adenomatous fibroadenomas), which all display intermediate to high signal intensity because of their high content of water and cells.

Finally, simple cysts can also be diagnosed quite reliably. They are characterized by regular borders, by homogeneous low signal intensity on T1-weighted images and homogeneous signal intensity on T2-weighted sequences, which increases with increasing T2-weighting.

Sanguinolent contents, in contrast, cause high signal intensity on T1-weighted sequences due to the paramagnetic properties of methemoglobin (80).

Criteria for a sufficient differentiation of the large number of other lesions and tissues, however, have been found neither on T2-weighted nor on T1-weighted SE sequences, nor on various gradient echo sequences such as FLASH or FISP (69). Instead, variable signal behavior with significant overlap of benign and malignant tissues has been encountered, which may be explained by the similar and quite variable composition of benign and malignant tissues.

Lately it has been reported that improved information by plain MRI may be possible through the additional use of a very strongly T1-weighted pulse sequence like STIR (127) or by systematic computer-aided evaluation of the signal intensities provided by a combined pulse sequence (32, 73), which consists of a selected T1- and T2-weighted and a so-called Dixon sequence. Since the latter studies (32, 73, 127) concern only a very small number of cases and thus a limited spectrum of pathology, more experience is needed to assess the value of the reported observations.

In summary, plain MRI of the breast has turned out to be more difficult than expected. Thus, it still must be considered investigational and should be used for diagnostic purposes only in carefully selected cases.

Contrast-enhanced MRI of the breast: principle and results

In view of the difficulties experienced with plain MRI, we started to investigate the use of Gd-DTPA (Magnevist®, Schering) for MRI of the breast in 1985. Gd-DTPA is the first paramagnetic contrast agent approved for clinical use in cranial and spinal MRI. It is under investigation for other indications of the body such as MRI of the breast. However, Gd—DTPA is not yet approved for this indication. It is excreted unchanged by glomerular filtration (serum half life about 90 minutes). The overall incidence of adverse events after intravenous injection of 0.1–0.2 mmol Gd-DTPA/kg body weight was found to be approximately 1%. Thus the tolerance is at least as good as that of iodinated nonionic X-ray contrast media. Especially the incidence of allergy-like reactions seems to be markedly lower than that of nonionic X-ray contrast media (95a). Fast bolus injections, if needed, are well tolerated (70a). In our personal experience we have seen no adverse events.

Our experience includes over 500 MRI studies of the breast with Gd-DTPA (38–42, 46, 48–54, 57–59). Since 1986, other groups have also started to work in this field (16, 66–70, 79, 82, 113, 117). Their results (which include approximately 500 additional cases) have confirmed and supplemented ours.

For contrast studies of the breast, the breast tissue is imaged with a T1-weighted pulse sequence once before and at least twice after the i.v. administration of Gd-DTPA. Due to the paramagnetic properties of Gd-DTPA, enhancing tissues are visualized as areas with signal increase on T1-weighted sequences.

For the final diagnosis the following features are taken into account:

– Amount of enhancement. Presence or absence of enhancement is determined by visual comparison of pre- and post-contrast slices. In addition, quantitative evaluation in regions of interest is possible.

– Pattern of enhancement. Focal enhancement can be described as irregularly shaped or well-circumscribed, lobulated, oval, or round. Diffuse enhancement of all or most of the breast tissue may be homogeneous or patchy.

– Speed of enhancement. It may roughly be estimated from the amount of enhancement on the first and second measurements after Gd-DTPA in the routine study. Dynamic studies make more exact evaluation possible.

The contrast behavior of the various lesions and tissue is described on pages 46–176.

In summary, all malignancies enhance significantly. Therefore absent enhancement very reliably excludes malignancy. However, some benign tissues or lesions also enhance depending on their amount of vascularity and interstitial space, but most of them only exhibit no or little enhancement. Delayed or diffuse enhancement favors the diagnosis of benignity, whereas focal and fast enhancement usually indicates lesions, which necessitate further work-up.

Thus contrast-enhanced MRI offers new, valuable information, which is based on differences of perfusion and interstitial space. It can and should be combined with information from conventional imaging. The application of contrast-enhanced MRI in diagnostically difficult cases and its value in the combined diagnostic approach together with other methods is discussed on pages 177-230.

Technique

In the female breast, very small tumors need to be detected and diagnosed. For this reason optimum technique is necessary in breast imaging.

In this chapter we point out the most important technical considerations necessary for high-quality contrast-enhanced MRI of the breast. Our own technique is described in detail for those interested in its application. Finally, possible future optimizations are mentioned.

Surface coil(s)

Surface coils had to be developed for MRI of the breast to obtain sufficient signal-to-noise (S/N) ratio (4, 116). The latter allows reduction of the slice thickness and improved resolution by direct zooming within acceptable imaging time.

Our experience shows that good coil sensitivity is just one factor of quality. It is, however, equally important to keep local variations in reception within the coil volume as low as possible. This is very important since strong local variations may cause the resulting signal intensity to be visually over- or underestimated.

Improved homogeneity can be achieved even for high-field magnets by the use of coils with several parallel windings (75). This construction is used in our breast coil for 1 Tesla. The quality of a coil can easily be tested by means of a big bottle filled with $CuSO_4$ solution, which is imaged within the coil. Inhomogeneities of the local reception are visualized as areas of increased or decreased signal intensity within one or several slices. Some increased amplification very close to the windings is normal. Figure 1 demonstrates the influence of locally inhomogeneous amplification.

For the diagnostic examination the patient should lie in the prone position on the breast coil. The pending breast(s) is (are) surrounded by the coil(s). Thus the anterior chest wall is in a fixed position and motion of the breast (with respiration) is usually minimal. Patient positioning on the single and double breast coil is shown in Figure 2.

Fig. 1   Surface coils

Figs. 1a–d
Inhomogeneities of reception.

Inhomogeneities of reception in different breast coils are visualized on images of a big bottle filled with CuSO$_4$ solution. Lines A and C indicate a vertical and horizontal line through the center of the coil. Line B indicates the upper margin of the coil (i.e., the level of the patient table). The usual position of the pending breast within the coil is also marked.

a) Phantom image, obtained with a preliminary first breast coil with one winding only. Very strong reception is visible close to the windings (arrows), whereas the reception at the bottom of the coil (X) is very poor.

b) Strong inhomogeneities within a breast image, obtained by the single winding coil (see a).

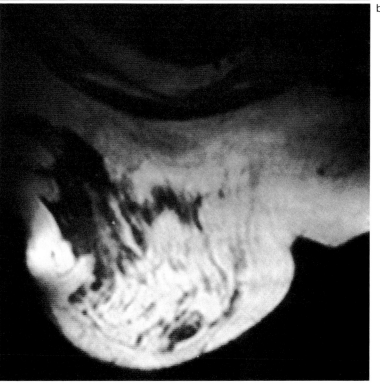

Fig. 1

c) Phantom image, obtained by our standard breast coil with 3 coil windings. Reception within the coil volume is much more homogeneous. Remaining inhomogeneities at the lateral margins (arrows) close to the windings are frequently not within the breast image. The overall lower reception at the bottom and upper margin of the coil have to be considered in quantitative evaluations (see normalization, page 31).

d) Phantom image of our double breast coil. It exhibits the most homogeneous reception, but a lower resolution (see page 24).

The windowing is identical in images a), c), and d) with reference to the maximum image intensity.

from (75)

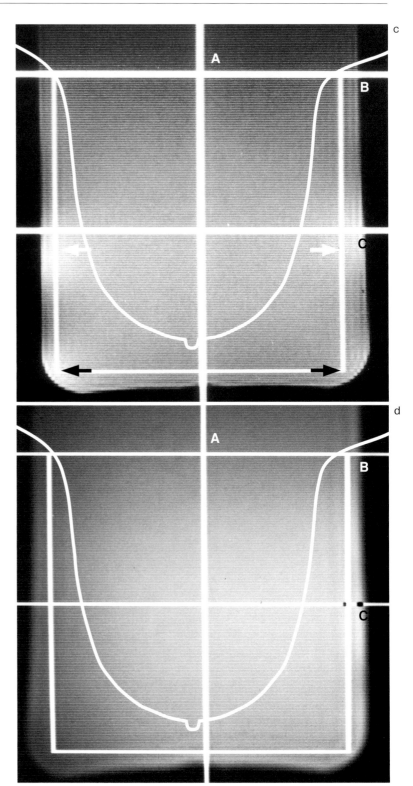

Fig. 2   Surface coils

Figs. 2a–d
Patient positioning.

a) Single breast coil: The patient lies on the table in a slightly oblique, prone position to allow optimum visualization of the axillary tail of the pending breast. The arm on the side of the examined breast is stretched. An infusion (NaCl 0.9%) is usually placed in the cubital vein of this arm. The infusion tube is then used to inject Gd-DTPA during the examination.

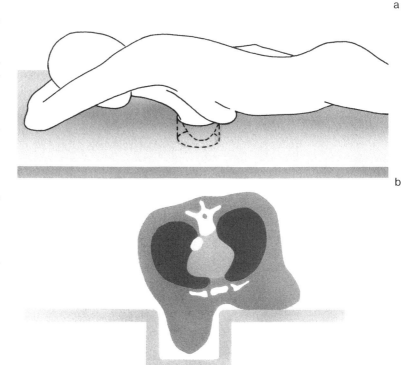

a

b

b) Schematic transverse slice through the patient demonstrates her position on the single breast coil.

c) Double breast coil: Here the patient usually lies in a straight prone position.

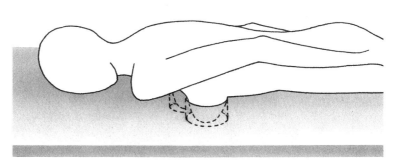

c

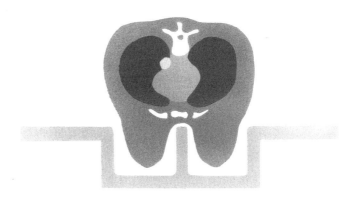

d) Schematic transverse slice through the patient demonstrates her position on the double breast coil.

d

We have predominantly used a single breast coil with a 21-cm field of view. It allows a resolution of about 0.8 mm (256·256 matrix, 1.4 gradient zoom) and excellent S/N ratio at slice thicknesses as low as 1-2 mm with a single acquisition at 1.0 Tesla. Slice thicknesses below 5 mm are obtained with 3D volume imaging.

For the great majority of our patients, the inner coil diameter of 15 cm proved sufficient. Very large breasts are usually quite fatty and can thus be excellently diagnosed by mammography alone. Furthermore, in very heavy patients the major limitation proved to be the opening of the magnet rather than the diameter of the breast coil.

Using double breast coils makes imaging of both breasts in one examination possible (15, 64, 67, 125). If, however, as in most presently available double breast coils, simultaneous imaging of both breasts is achieved by a larger field of view, lower resolution, impossibility of zooming (because of aliasing artifacts), and decreased S/N ratio are significant disadvantages.

Therefore, double breast coils that allow sequential (instead of simultaneous) imaging of both breasts with off-center zoom are preferable, since only thus can the same resolution be achieved as with the single breast coil. For lesions in the axillary tail a single breast coil is still better suited, since the axillary tail is best included within the coil volume when the patient turns slightly to the side in the prone position. Optimizations such as further extension of lateral coil windings toward the chest wall might improve reception within the axillary tail in double breast coils. Double breast coils allow the useful imaging of both breasts and thus will probably become more and more important. However, specific further technical improvements are needed to achieve same image quality and information as presently available with single breast coils.

Course of examination and choice of pulse sequence

General requirements

In our opinion a standard technique has to fulfill several requirements:

● Evaluation of the complete breast tissue must be guaranteed. When only selected slices are imaged, a negative MRI examination can never exclude the presence of a lesion.

● Short measurement time is necessary to avoid patient motion due to the uncomfortable position. Dynamic studies prove that the discrimination between lesion and surrounding tissue is best during the first 5 minutes postinjection of Gd-DTPA. For this reason a technique should be chosen that allows imaging of the complete breast tissue within about 5 minutes.

● Optimum image quality and maximum signal increase in enhancing areas should be attempted. For adequate visualization of small lesions a resolution of 1 mm or less appears necessary.

In addition, because of possible partial volume effect, detectability of very small enhancing lesions depends on the relation of lesion size and slice thickness used and – very important – on the relative signal increase caused by Gd-DTPA. The latter is determined by the sensitivity of the pulse sequence for Gd-DTPA and by the dosage of Gd-DTPA, which is administered intravenously.

According to our experience, slice thickness should not exceed 5 mm. Very thin contiguous slices (1 mm) avoid significant partial volume effect, but the number of slices per breast examination increases drastically (100 images for a breast thickness of 10 cm!) as does measurement time (at least 10 minutes per sequence even with 3D fast imaging).

The most sensitive pulse sequences for Gd-DTPA have so far been gradient echo fast imaging sequences (FI) (e.g., FLASH). The dosage of Gd-DTPA, which depends on the pulse sequence used, can be lower for the very sensitive FI sequences (0.1-0.16 mmol/kg) than for SE sequences (0.2 mmol/kg).

● The technique should be as simple as possible to ensure identical measurement conditions and thus good reproducibility.

● The user should have sufficient experience (knowledge of artifacts, knowledge of the thresholds for significant enhancement) before using a technique clinically.

Based on our experience since 1984, we have developed the following standard technique:

● Before positioning the patient, an infusion (NaCl 0.9%) is placed into the cubital vein of the arm beside the breast that is to be examined. The infusion tube is later used to administer Gd-DTPA during the examination.

● The patient is examined in the prone position. She lies on top of the breast coil which surrounds her breast.

The most comfortable position for examining one breast appears to be a slightly oblique prone position with one arm elevated (to support the head) and the arm on the side of the breast in question stretched beside the body. That way the patient may turn slightly to the side, which seems to be more comfortable for patients with degenerative changes of the cervical spine (Figs. 2a and b).

For imaging of both breasts with the double breast coil the patient should, of course, lie in the straight prone position. The head is supported by a small cushion. Both arms are beside the body (Figs. 2c and d).

When the patient is positioned on top of the coil, exact horizontal orientation of the coil must be checked. To avoid slipping and angling of the coil on the table we have attached an antislip layer to the bottom of our coil.

● The patient is then moved into the magnet and after the necessary adjustment the complete breast is imaged once before and twice after (minutes 0–5 and 7–12 postcontrast) the application of Gd-DTPA. The first postcontrast measurement shows early enhancement, whereas the second detects delayed enhancement. Both postcontrast pulse sequences together allow a rough assessment of the speed of enhancement.

● For contrast studies of the breast we have chosen a 3D FLASH sequence, which offers several advantages (59):

– Compared to 2D imaging (as used for SE sequences) 3D techniques allow a significantly better S/N ratio.

– With 3D technique all slices are imaged simultaneously. With 2D technique, so far at least two measurements were necessary to image the complete breast. Thus with 3D technique the enhancement of all slices is averaged over the first 5 minutes (first postcontrast measurement) or over minutes 7-12 (second postcontrast measurement). This technique allows exact comparison of the enhancement in all slices.

– The short measurement time necessary for imaging all slices is especially advantageous for the postcontrast measurement, since for most lesions discrimination is best during the first 5 minutes.

– Because of the very high sensitivity of FLASH for Gd-DTPA, enhancing areas assume very high signal intensity and thus become quite obvious.

– The signal intensity of fat with FLASH is usually smaller than the signal intensity of enhancing areas. Therefore confusion of enhancing areas and fat is far less likely with FLASH than with SE sequences. In the latter, fat displays intermediate to high signal intensity, whereas enhancement usually assumes only intermediate signal intensity (Fig. 3). This is especially important if patient motion (and thus changing partial volume of fat) occurs.

With our first imager (Magnetom M 10, Siemens, installed in 1984, upgraded to 1.0 Tesla in 1985) the following pulse sequence has proven optimum and has been used since 1987: FLASH 3D: TR = 40 ms, TE = 14 ms, FA = 50°, imaging volume 10–12 cm, 32 slices, slice thickness 3–4 mm, direct zoom 1.4, 1 acquisition, measurement time 5 minutes, calculation time 2 minutes.

Further optimizations have now become possible with the latest equipment (Magnetom 63 SP, Siemens, 1.5 Tesla, installed in 1990): Shorter TE allows shortening of TR, reduction of motion artifacts, and slightly stronger T1-weighting.

Shortening of TR (to about 20 ms) can be used to further reduce measurement time (e.g., FLASH 3D: TR = 20 ms, TE = 6 ms, FA = 50°–90°, 32 slices, measurement time 2–3 minutes). Thus, with the shorter measurement time, the complete breast tissue can be imaged at even shorter intervals post contrast medium.

Reduction of TR can also be used to further decrease the slice thickness and thus the influence of partial volume effects (e.g., FLASH 3D: TR = 20 ms, TE = 5 ms, FA = 50°–90°, 64 slices, slice thickness < 2 mm, 1 acquisition, measurement time 5 minutes). This can be useful for assessing very small lesions.

With the new possibilities one should, however, consider that reduction of slice thickness significantly increases the number of images to be evaluated per breast.

● Present overall measurement time (including the 3D FLASH sequences, patient positioning and adjustments) does not exceed 30 to 40 minutes. The time factor should also be considered for other techniques, since motion between the measurements (from uncomfortable positioning or long examination time) complicates the following evaluation; motion during the measurements degrades image quality.

● During the study, optimum elimination of the following artifacts is required (see also Fig. 4):

– Artifacts, which may appear at the border of the imaging volume in 3D technique due to aliasing, can be avoided by choosing a volume somewhat larger than the breast.

– To avoid potential artifacts caused by direct skin contact, the paper towel on the examination table should also cover the inside of the breast coil.

– Severe artifacts that may be caused by angling or slipping of the coil can be avoided by attaching an antislip layer to the bottom of the coil.

– Respiratory motion artifacts are quite well eliminated if the patient is examined in the prone position.

– Most important is the elimination of motion artifacts caused by the heart. They usually cross the left breast and sometimes even the medial parts of the right breast.

With our equipment, this can be avoided only by switching phase and frequency encoding gradients*. Thus the artifacts can be turned 90° and then usually cross above the breast horizontally. Artifacts in this position may, however, cause problems in detecting lesions in the outer axillary tail. Here, it may be wise either not to switch the gradients or to turn the patient slightly further to the side, so that the horizontally running artifacts do not cross the tissue in question.

* EKG-gating has not proven useful due to incomplete elimination of the motion artifacts and prolonged examination time.

If the gradients have to be switched (with our present software and hardware), the frequency filter of the receiver must be adapted, because of the eccentric position of the breast in the magnet and the small field of view. Otherwise part of the breast may be "cut off" and not imaged. Therefore the MRI breast study is slightly more complicated than other examinations.

An easier solution of the problem of heart motion, which has now become possible with the latest equipment, is local presaturation of the region of heart.

– Finally, severe diagnostic problems may occur with data overflow. Such images are characterized by a higher background signal intensity (sometimes wavelike) and should – even though they are not distorted – by no means be interpreted, since significant changes of contrast have been encountered in all or only part of the image (see Fig. 3). Data overflow may occur, for example when ferromagnetic metal is left on the patient (sometimes only a tiny zipper!).

● Gd-DTPA is applied intravenously through the existing infusion tube. We inject the complete dosage within about 1 minute. This injection is followed by another injection of 20 ml NaCl 0.9% (to empty the tube). The dosage of Gd-DTPA depends on the pulse sequence used. For T1-weighted SE imaging (see below) a dosage of 0.2 mmol/kg body weight is necessary (48). This dosage can be reduced if FLASH sequences are used, because of their excellent sensitivity to Gd-DTPA. We recommend a dosage of 0.16 mmol/kg body weight (with this dosage the volume injected in ml is one third of the body weight, e.g., 20 ml for 60 kg body weight), since we do not want to risk the excellent detectability of very small lesions. Whether a further reduction to 0.1 mmol/kg, as applied by Kaiser (70), leads to equivalent results in all cases, is still being investigated in a comparative study.

● Evaluation of the study is then performed visually and, if necessary (see page 46), quantitatively. For the visual evaluation pre- and postcontrast images are compared slice by slice to search for areas with signal increase. Such an exact comparison is necessary because of the very variable composition of breast tissue of high-signal-intensity fat lobules and low-signal-intensity glandular tissues. Even though enhancement is visible on both SE and FLASH sequences, the recognition of small enhancing areas on FLASH pulse sequences (with 0.16 mmol Gd-DTPA/kg) (see Fig. 65) is much easier and thus safer than on SE sequences (compare Fig. 31). This is due to the prominent signal increase of enhancing areas and the relatively lower signal intensity of fat on FLASH sequences.

A careful choice of window setting is an important requirement for exact visual evaluation. The window must be wide enough to allow good distinction between the high-signal-intensity enhancing areas and fat lobules (important for FLASH), but the window must be narrow enough to show less prominent signal increase (very important for SE). If with the narrow window necessary for SE imaging breast tissue outside the coil cannot be assessed adequately, it is necessary to evaluate the tissue outside the coil separately with a similar or even narrower window, but a different center.

We have had good experience with the following window settings:

– For SE sequences, the window width should exceed the maximum image signal intensity, measured within fat, by no more than 30%.

– For FLASH images, a window width of about 3 times the signal intensity of fat has proven useful.

– After the window is adapted a center is chosen that best shows all tissues after Gd-DTPA.

– Pre- and postcontrast scans are photographed with the same window setting.

In breasts consisting of numerous small lobules of fat and glandular tissue, visual evaluation can be supported by subtraction (or even better division) of the corresponding post- and precontrast slices (see Figs. 31 and 68). Division also eliminates those visual differences of signal increase caused by locally different coil reception, since the locally different amplification factor is thus dropped. Provided no significant motion occurs between the measurements, which is the case in about 90% of our examinations, the subtraction (or division) images show signal increase only within enhancing areas and blood vessels. Motion is indicated by the appearance of rimlike subtraction lines at the borders of the breast as well as at the interfaces between fatty and glandular tissue.

A quantitative evaluation is useful in cases of borderline enhancement and can be performed in regions of interest. For this quantitative evaluation, a normalization is necessary. It takes into account local variations of the reception, caused by the geometry of the breast coil, and varying adjustment in different patients.

For our evaluations, we have used the following method:

First the signal increase (in units of image signal intensity) is measured within the area in question (e.g., 200 units). Then the local signal intensity of fat adjacent to this area (e.g., 500 units) is measured. Then the multiplication factor necessary to obtain a signal intensity of 1500 "normalized units" (NU) in this adjacent fat is determined (e.g., 1500:500 = 3). The normalized signal increase in the area in question (in NU) results from its measured signal increase multiplied by the normalization factor (e.g., 200 NU $\cdot$ 3 = 600 NU).

Other possibilities and special techniques

SE sequences

With some equipment FLASH 3D imaging is not yet possible. Then T1-weighted SE sequences, which we used until 1987, can be applied instead. The shortest possible echo times should be chosen to obtain optimal T1-weighting and to allow simultaneous measurement of as many slices as possible. Even though 3D imaging is not possible with these SE sequences, the complete breast can in general be imaged within about 5 to 6 minutes by two T1-weighted SE sequences with 5 mm slice thickness (e.g., SE: TR = 500–600 ms, TE = 17 ms, 10–12 slices, 5 mm slice thickness, 1 acquisition, 1.0 Tesla). Due to the lower S/N ratio obtainable with this 2D technique, the larger slice thickness, the high signal intensity of fat, which may pose problems in case of partial volume and patient motion, and the lower sensitivity for Gd-DTPA, the recognition of small enhancing areas may be limited.

For these reasons a higher dosage of Gd-DTPA (0.2 mmol/kg) should be used, and evaluation must very carefully consider even slight changes of signal intensity at a narrow window setting.

Dynamic contrast studies

This method (53, 54, 58, 113), which has lately been favored by others investigators (68, 70), is interesting for specific research purposes.

To study the course of enhancement in certain tissues, selected slices are imaged before and repeatedly after the i.v. administration of Gd-DTPA by 2D FLASH (TR = 40–200 ms, TE = 5–14 ms depending on the equipment, FA = 50°–90°, 1–7 slices).

To improve reproducibility several standardizations are necessary: Injection into cubital vein only (injection of the contrast medium* within 1 minute followed by injection of NaCl), exact timing of both injection and start of measurement.

For fundamental studies, the method offers interesting aspects, both concerning general understanding and discrimination of lesions, as will also be shown on page 49. However, because of similar speed of enhancement of some benign and malignant lesions, this method cannot be considered a completely reliable tool for diagnostic purposes. In particular, it does not allow to exclude malignancy (see pages 49, 104) based on a delayed enhancement only, since late enhancement has proven a rare feature of a few carcinomas.

If this method is used diagnostically, another drawback is the fact that presently only a certain number of slices, which have to be selected before contrast medium is applied, can be examined. Therefore, if no enhancement is seen, the risk remains that the lesion in question was not included.

For these reasons this technique appears to us an interesting additional method if further information is desired. But as long as the complete breast tissue is not imaged we cannot recommend it for a routine study.

* Dosage see page 29.

*Pulse sequences that allow suppression
of fat signal*

Interpretation of contrast-enhanced MRI of the breast may be complicated by individually varying amounts of interposed fat lobules. For this reason, an exact visual comparison of the corresponding pre- and postcontrast slices is necessary to distinguish enhancing areas (with low signal intensity before contrast material) from fat lobules (which display high signal intensity on pre- and postcontrast scans).

The problem has been alleviated significantly since the introduction of FLASH imaging, because (with these sequences and a sufficient dosage* of Gd-DTPA) even small enhancing areas usually assume higher signal intensities than fat. Another significant aid is offered by subtraction or better division images of the corresponding post- and precontrast slices, provided the patient has not moved between the measurements.

However, even further improvement of visibility and interpretation of enhancement can be expected from pulse sequences, which allow direct suppression of fat signal. Several sequences are presently under investigation for this purpose: CHESS or similar sequences (19, 20) and PEACH (118).

CHESS or similar sequences are based on a gradient-echo fast-imaging pulse sequence. Either the fat signal is eliminated by a presaturation pulse or the water signal is excited selectively. Provided the equipment allows fast (automatic) shimming, short measurement time and the possibility of 3D acquisition are major advantages.

PEACH is based on an SE type sequence and – as a so-called hybrid method – uses both the Dixon method and a presaturation pulse to eliminate the fat signal. The method presently only allows 2D acquisition.

Figure 5 shows various "fat" and "water" images. Since so far for these techniques sequence tuning and shimming are quite complicated and critical and therefore prone to error, further research remains necessary.

*Special technique for preoperative marking
of breast lesions*

Even though at our institution MRI is used chiefly to solve diagnostic problems, several additional nonpalpable lesions, which were not visualized by other methods, have so far been

* Dosage see page 29.

detected by MRI. For these cases an MRI marking technique that helps to guide biopsy must be offered, because according to our experience biopsy of any lesion based on the routine MRI study alone cannot be recommended. The reason is that the routine MRI examination is performed in the prone position, whereas biopsy has to be performed in the supine position. Some lesions, however, "move" significantly – especially in the longitudinal direction – when position is changed. In other words, lesions that were imaged in the lower quadrant in the prone position may be imaged in the upper quadrant in the supine position and vice versa (compare Figs. 64 and 72).

Therefore we have developed the following technique* (42), in which the patient is reexamined in the supine position and the lesion is subsequently marked by direct injection of a charcoal/Gd-DTPA mixture into the pathologic tissue: To obtain a sufficient S/N ratio without the usual breast coil, a simple surface coil or Helmholtz-type coil can be used. With the Helmholtz coil, direct zooming is not possible, since it might cause superimposition of the spine and parts of the breast tissue.

After an infusion tube is placed, the patient is asked to lie down on the examination table, this time in the supine position with her arms beside her body. Then the breast is strapped to the chest wall as tightly as possible by several stripes of white tape, that run around the anterior chest wall. The breast is covered with a sheet of paper towel and the coil is positioned above the breast. Before the patient is completely moved into the magnet, the center of the imaging volume (slice position zero) is marked on the patient with a pen by means of the laser cross on the MRI unit. Then the examination is started, consisting of one FLASH 3D pulse sequence before and one FLASH 3D pulse sequence after the i.v. administration of 0.16–0.2 mmol Gd-DTPA/kg. The higher dosage of 0.2 mmol/kg is especially recommended for very small lesions, since compared to the standard examination the images are usually somewhat blurred by increased respiratory motion of the breast in the supine position (see Fig. 6). Therefore exact comparison of pre- and postcontrast slices is advisable.

* Note: This technique is not part of the officially approved recommendations for dosage and application mode of Gd-DTPA.

After the lesion is recognized, its exact position relative to the center of the imaging volume is determined by its coordinates within the image and by its slice position. Its depth from the skin surface can also be measured within the image. This localization technique is the same as usually applied for CT-guided biopsy. In general, we insert the needle into the breast in an exact vertical direction (pointing toward the table). If the needle would thus cross the nipple or areola, it can be angled or inserted horizontally instead after the appropriate measurements are taken from the image. An ordinary 20-gauge metal needle usually serves this purpose. If check of the needle position is desired before the area is marked (e.g., in case of patient motion), a special nonmagnetic 20-gauge needle can also be used (81), which allows imaging of the breast with the needle in place.

Then the following mixture is injected directly into the pathologic tissue through the needle:
1–1.5 ml charcoal suspension 4% in 0.9% NaCl and 0.1–0.15 ml Gd-DTPA 0.5 mmol/ml.

Finally the complete breast is imaged once more to confirm correct position of the mixture. Due to the high concentration of Gd-DTPA, a signal loss is visible in the center of the injected area. At the borders, where Gd-DTPA starts to distribute, a rimlike enhancement is visible (see Fig. 6).

The charcoal suspension itself does not distribute further. Thus it remains within the area in question until it is detected and removed by the surgeon. The major advantage of this suspension compared to methylene blue is that it eliminates the need for exact timing of MRI examination and operation. If operation within 1 to 2 hours after the marking is possible, 1–1.5 ml charcoal suspension can be replaced by 1 ml charcoal suspension and 0.5 ml methylene blue. The advantage of methylene blue is that it distributes in a broader area and can thus be found more easily by the surgeon. Charcoal helps the pathologist to find small suspicious areas, since it does not distribute.

Our experience shows that quite exact marking is possible ($\pm$5 to 10 mm) with this technique, provided the lesion can be well identified. Due to the increased blurring by respiratory motion in the supine position this method might not allow to identify very small lesions. Therefore further improvement of the marking technique is still desirable.

Fig. 3

Figs. 3a–f
Comparison of FLASH 3D and SE technique in a patient with interesting mammographic findings (no palpable abnormality).

a) This only previous mammogram (mediolateral view) from 6 years before had demonstrated very fine indeterminate to suspicious microcalcifications within major parts of the breast tissue. Biopsy at that time had revealed proliferative dysplasia.

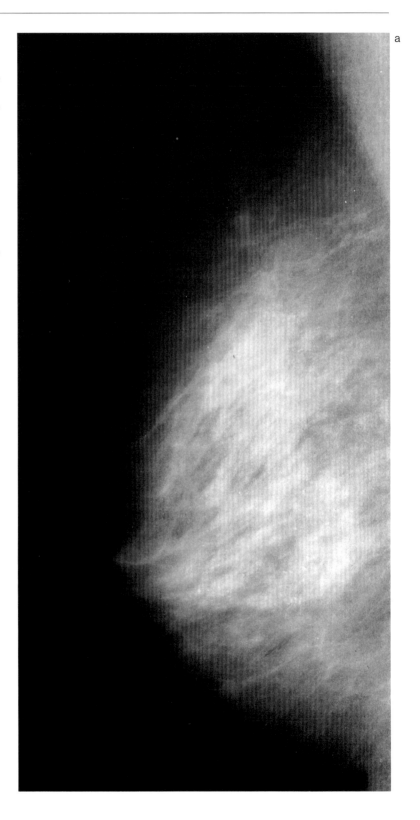

a

Fig. 3   Technique

b) The mammogram at presentation now showed persisting indeterminate microcalcifications. Their decrease in number is explained by the biopsy performed after the first mammogram. MRI was performed because of contradicting opinions of several radiologists concerning recommendation of a second biopsy.

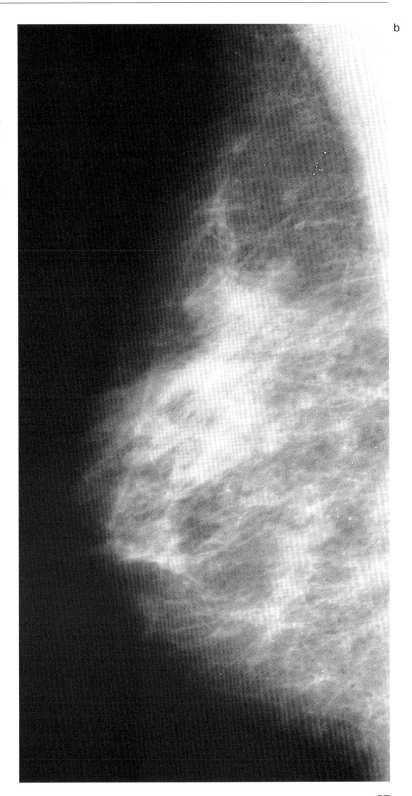

b

Fig. 3

c) FLASH 3D precontrast image (TR = 40 ms, TE = 14 ms, FA = 50°, one of 32 images acquired in 5 minutes). Fat displays intermediate signal intensity, the remaining tissue low signal intensity.

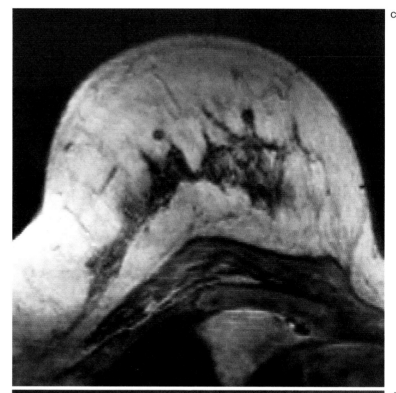

c

d) FLASH 3D postcontrast image (same slice, same pulse sequence). Significant enhancement (arrows), which due to its strong signal increase is quite obvious, is seen within large parts of the tissue and within the vessels (v).

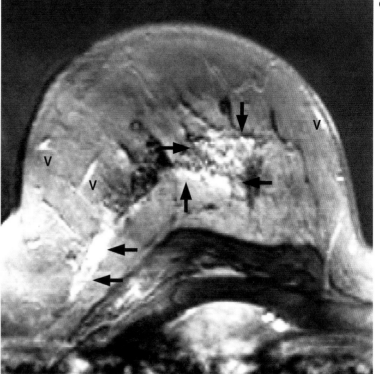

d

Fig. 3

Technique

e) Precontrast SE image (TR = 0.5 sec, TE = 17 ms). Compared to c), the signal intensity of fat is much stronger.

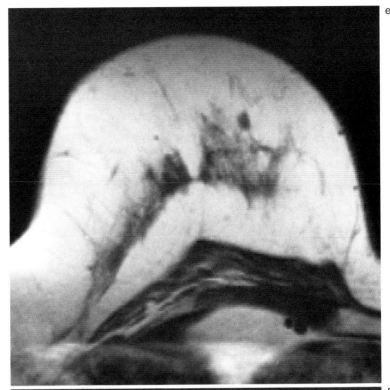

e

f) Postcontrast SE image (same slice, same pulse sequence). Here enhancing areas within the tissue are visible by their signal increase (arrows) compared to the precontrast image, but they are less obvious than with the FLASH sequence.

Histology: the enhancing areas corresponded to an extensive intraductally growing carcinoma.

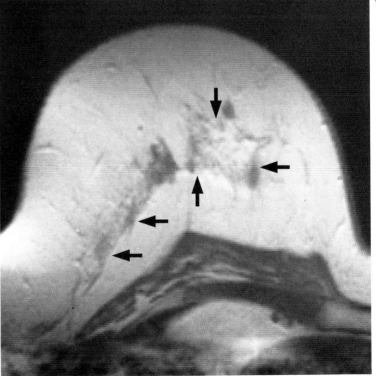

f

Fig. 4

Figs. 4a–c
Various artifacts.

a, b) A case is shown in which artifacts of unknown origin were the cause of severe misinterpretation: In this patient with mammographically dense tissue and positive axillary lymph nodes, contrast-enhanced MRI was performed, since malignancy could neither be identified nor completely excluded by mammography, sonography and palpation.

a) On the good-quality precontrast image, dense breast tissue includes two areas with very low signal intensity, which in retrospect probably correspond to signal voids.

b) On the postcontrast image, a ringlike strong signal intensity was seen around these two low signal intensity areas. Since this high signal intensity was not present on the precontrast images, it was interpreted as ringlike enhancement within the wall of centrally necrotic tumors (compare with Fig. 49). This interpretation even matched with the fact that the patient had undergone several courses of chemotherapy before MRI. Thus MR-guided biopsy was recommended. The wavelike artifacts on the postcontrast image had at that time been noted but had not been considered important.

Histologically, however, no tumor and no necrosis was found.
Instead, old scarring was seen. It was caused by an operation several years ago, which was no longer visible on the skin and which the patient had not considered important enough to mention. Thus, in retrospect both the

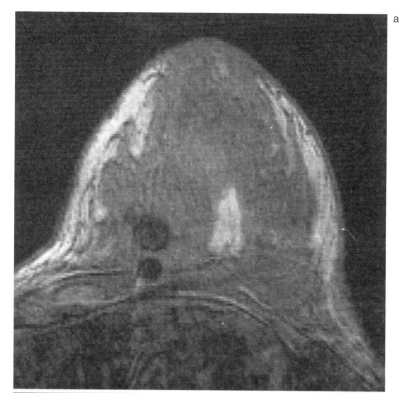

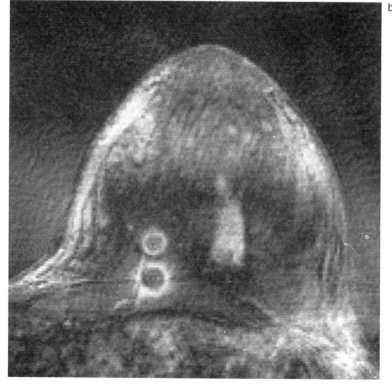

Fig. 4   Technique

signal void (a) and the ringlike increased signal intensity around the signal void (b) are probably caused by some kind of metallic artifacts, possibly residual glove powder. The unusual appearance on the postcontrast image could be explained by data overflow, which became more prominent after i.v. injection of Gd-DTPA. This is also supported by the varying and increased background signal intensity.

This case is illustrated to warn against any interpretation of images containing artifacts.

c) Another case with wavelike artifacts. Such artifacts might be caused by folding.

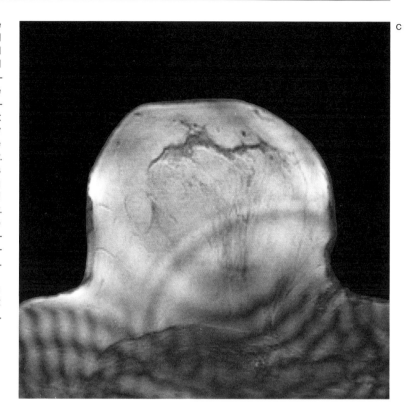

c

Fig. 5

Figs. 5a–d
Fat/water separation.

The effect of selective imaging of fat and water protons is shown in these images of a normal volunteer as well as of a small tube (t) filled with a solution of Gd-DTPA (2 mmol Gd-DTPA/ liter water).
a) On the "fat" image only the fat is visualized. It surrounds the glandular tissue. No signal is received from the glandular tissue or the tube, since neither of them contains fat protons. The shown image is one of 64 slices of a 3D fast imaging gradient echo pulse sequence with spectral selective excitation of the fat component by a 1–3–3–1 pulse; TR=23 ms, TE=9 ms, FA=50°, slice thickness 1.2 mm, 1 acquisition, measurement time: 6 minutes. The plane of the reconstruction of c) is indicated by line A.

b) On the "water" image no signal is received from fat. Glandular tissue exhibits low to intermediate signal intensity. With stronger T1-weighting its signal intensity could even be further decreased. The very strong signal received from the solution in the very small tube (t) (cross section) is caused by the T1-shortening by Gd-DTPA and represents the enhancement seen in vessels or lesions after i.v. injection of Gd-DTPA. The shown image is one of 64 slices of a fast imaging gradient echo pulse sequence with spectral selective excitation of the water component by a 1–3–3–1 pulse; TR = 23 ms, TE = 9 ms, FA = 50°, slice thickness 1.2 mm, 1 acquisition, measurement time: 6 minutes. The plane of the reconstruction of d) is indicated by line B.

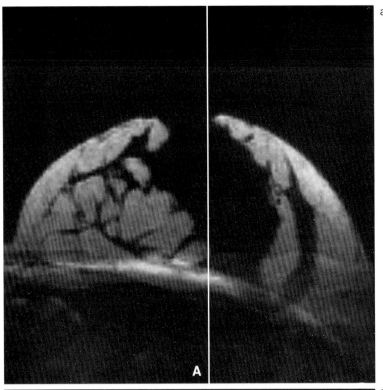

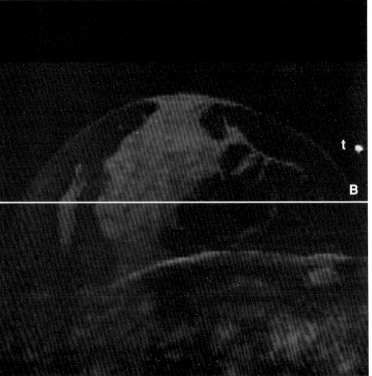

Fig. 5   Technique

With slice thicknesses of 1–2 mm, as used in this case, excellent image quality is also obtained, when other planes are reconstructed using this 3D data set. Such reconstructions might be helpful to better assess the exact configuration, extension and localization of a lesion.

c) Sagittal reconstructed image of the central section of the breast showing the fat component only. The arrowheads point to an artifact caused by the small size of the selected volume. (C = chest wall, N = nipple area)

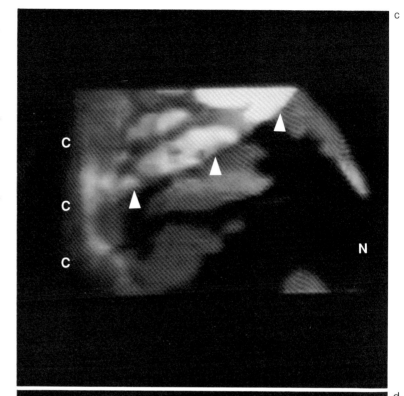

d) Reconstructed frontal image of the scanned breast tissue showing the water component only. (G = glandular tissue, S = skin surface)

Images from Dr. M. Deimling and Dr. G. Decke, Siemens AG.

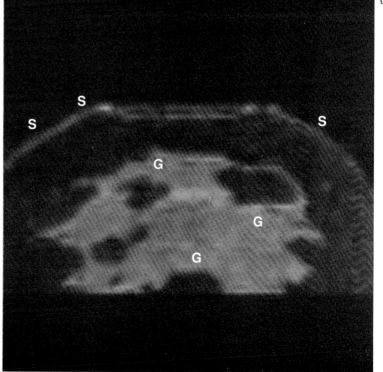

Fig. 6

Figs. 6a–d
MR-guided needle localization of a suspicious area. In this patient with a mammographically very dense breast and clinically very lumpy breast, a questionable hypoechoic area had been detected sonographically. Because of the uncertain sonographic findings with impossible clinical correlation even in retrospect, MRI was performed.

a) Precontrast image (FLASH 3D: TR = 40 ms, TE = 14 ms, FA = 50°, one of 32 slices acquired in 5 minutes).

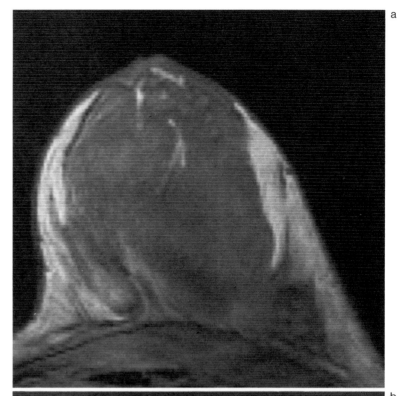

b) Postcontrast image (same slice, same pulse sequence). A highly suspicious irregular area of focal strong contrast enhancement (arrow) is identified in this routine study obtained with the patient in the prone position on the breast coil.

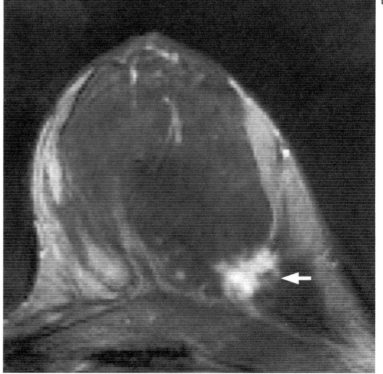

Fig. 6   Technique

c) The postcontrast image of a repeated contrast study directly before needle localization. It was acquired directly after injection of 0.2 mmol Gd-DTPA/kg (higher dosage) with the same pulse sequence as b), but using the Helmholtz coil and with the patient in the supine position. Since in the supine position the outer parts of the breast in particular are situated more laterally, the gradients have not been switched, and motion artifacts cross the medial parts of the breast. Compared to b), the area of enhancement is less distinct because of the lower resolution (Helmholtz coil) and – most important – respiratory motion. Position of the suspicious area is indicated by the slice position, by its distance from the y-axis (d1) (laser), and by its depth under the skin surface (d2).

d) The same area is imaged again with the same pulse sequence after direct injection of marking solution (charcoal and Gd-DTPA) into the suspicious area. The marking solution causes a central signal void surrounded by a rim of increased signal intensity (arrows).

Histology: ductal carcinoma.

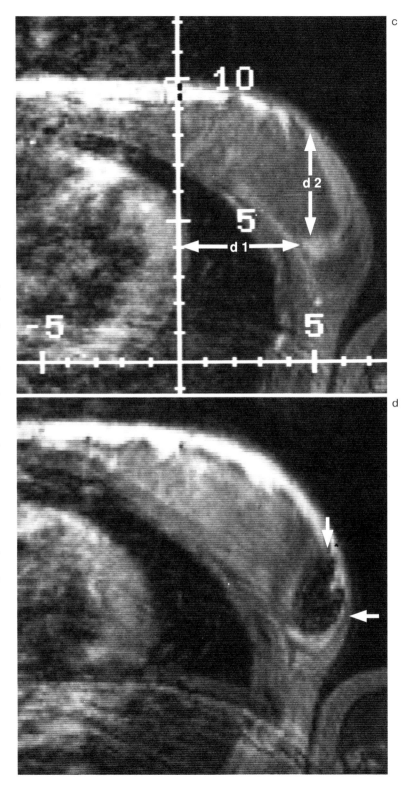

Appearance of various tissues and lesions

General aspects

Pages 51–176 treat the various pathologies in detail, this section provides the reader with a general outline for the interpretation of MRI studies of the breast.

The results presented in this book are based on the data from over 500 MRI examinations of the breast performed with Gd-DTPA at our institution. Worldwide experience, which includes almost another 500 cases, is considered as well. For quantitative results, only measurements from our biopsy-proven cases (Tables 1–8) were used.

All our cases have been evaluated qualitatively and quantitatively using the standard technique (pages 26–31) and sometimes further studies (dynamic measurements or different pulse sequences for comparison). For most routine cases qualitative evaluation of the standard examination appears sufficient. We do recommend quantitative evaluation of the amount of enhancement (page 31) for all borderline cases, where enhancement is not easily classified as significant or nonsignificant and for the first 50 to 100 cases to gain the necessary experience and threshold data. The quantitative evaluation helps to avoid mistakes caused by too wide or narrow window settings or by quality changes of the coil reception during the measurement (technical problems). Furthermore, the threshold for significance of enhancement needs to be checked, since it depends on the equipment used, the pulse sequences, the dosage of Gd-DTPA and the normalization. The threshold for significance must be below the value of the mean signal increase in carcinomas minus at least its double standard deviation.

In our case, these considerations yielded a threshold of 200–250 normalized units (NU) for SE technique (dosage of Gd-DTPA: 0.2 mmol/kg) and a threshold of 500 NU for 3D fast-imaging technique (0.16 mmol Gd-DTPA/kg). So far enhancement in all carcinomas was > 280 NU on SE imaging and > 700 NU on FLASH imaging (FI).

In the evaluation of contrast-enhanced MR images of the breast three predominant features make up the appearance of various lesions and tissues: amount, pattern, and speed of enhancement.

Amount of enhancement is the most important information. It is assessed visually and, if necessary, measured quantitatively. Table 1 gives an overview of the amount of signal increase measured after Gd-DTPA with SE and 3D fast imaging. As shown, normal breast tissue, nonproliferative dysplasia, and old scarring usually enhance insignificantly. Significant enhancement occurred in all carcinomas and in the majority of benign tumors (fibroadenomas, papillomas). Variable enhancement is seen in proliferative dysplasias and inflammatory changes, including fresh postoperative or postradiation changes (see pages 138-176). Since all carcinomas enhance significantly, insignificance or absence of enhancement has proven a most valuable piece of information. In fact, insignificant enhancement is so far the only reliable criterion for exclusion of malignancy. Of course, this criterion can only be used for lesions larger than slice thickness (partial volume effect), which is counterchecked against the other methods. In case of significant enhancement, pattern and speed of the enhancement are considered as well.

Pattern of enhancement is the second important feature. We predominantly distinguish focal from diffuse enhancement (Table 2). In case of focal enhancement, the chance of detecting a previously unknown malignancy (e.g., within dense tissue) exists because of the very high sensitivity of MRI for all enhancing lesions (100% sensitivity for carcinomas so far). Since focal enhancement can be caused by several lesions, usually benign and malignant tumors, sometimes focal proliferative dysplasia and rarely other lesions, the sensitivity is, of course, higher than the specificity of such findings (see pages 177–180, Tables 10, 11).

As is known from mammography, irregular contours favor a diagnosis of malignancy. The major differential diagnoses to be considered in presence of irregular contours are carcinoma > focal proliferative dysplasia > benign tumor with irregular outlines > rare focal inflammatory lesion or fat necrosis. Well-circumscribed outlines favor a diagnosis of benign lesion. Here the differential diagnoses are fibroadenoma or papilloma > focal proliferative dysplasia > well-circumscribed malignancy (see also page 77). It should, however, be emphasized that – as is known from the other modalities – the

Table 1
Amount of enhancement measured in 377 biopsy-proven tissues and lesions.

Amount of enhancement is indicated as mean ± single standard deviation of the signal increase measured in normalized units (NU) after injection of 0.16 mmol Gd-DTPA/kg.

The numbers in brackets indicate the number of tissues measured with each technique. Since some tissues have been examined by more than one technique, the sum of the numbers in brackets is equal or higher than the number of cases examined.

The absolute amount of enhancement and the thresholds are valid for our standard technique. They depend on the equipment, the pulse sequences, the normalization and the dosage of Gd-DTPA.

tissue or lesion	no. of cases examined	amount of enhancement		
		2D SE technique 0.35 Tesla	2D SE technique 1.0 Tesla	3D FLASH technique 1.0 Tesla
carcinoma	131	458±103 (n=28)	526±155 (n=77)	1125±277 (n=43)
lymphoma	2	–	–	735±55 (n=2)
cystosarcoma	1	–	–	2500 (n=1)
fibroadenoma	38	528±150 (n=6)	608±277 (n=27)	1295±641 (n=10)
papilloma	3	–	350 (n=1)	833±490 (n=3)
nonproliferative dysplasia and normal breast tissue	91	120±51 (n=12)	122±80 (n=55)	95±97 (n=43)
proliferative dysplasia (including moderate and strong proliferative dysplasia and adenosis)	91	245±67 (n=16)	402±165 (n=58)	687±325 (n=28)
scarring (fresh) and fat necrosis	6	–	403±93 (n=5)	1180±150 (n=2)
scarring (old)	8	140±40 (n=2)	118±44 (n=5)	144±60 (n=4)
inflammation	7	390 (n=1)	452±180 (n=5)	418 (n=1)
threshold of significance		250	200–250	500

presence of well-circumscribed contours of round or oval shape are not completely certain criteria for the exclusion of malignancy.

Diffuse enhancement describes either homogeneous or patchy enhancement of all or large parts of the breast tissue. This type of enhancement unfortunately has proven quite uncharacteristic, since it may be caused both by benign (most frequently) and malignant changes (less frequently). The differential diagnosis of diffusely enhancing tissues includes, with decreasing likelihood, proliferative dysplasias > secretory disease > inflammatory and post-therapeutic changes > diffusely growing malignancies.

Table 2
Pattern of enhancement
in 377 biopsy-proven
tissues and lesions.

tissue or lesion	no. of cases examined	pattern of enhancement			
		no enhance-ment	focal enhance-ment: round	focal enhance-ment: irregular	diffuse enhance-ment
carcinoma	131	0	12	101	18
lymphoma	2	0	1	1	0
cystosarcoma	1	0	1	0	0
fibroadenoma	38	2	27	7	2
papilloma	3	1	2	0	0
nonproliferative dysplasia and normal breast tissue	91	87	0	0	4
proliferative dysplasia (including moderate and strong proliferative dysplasia and adenosis)	91	9	0	12	70
scarring (fresh) and fat necrosis	6	0	1	4	1
scarring (old)	8	8	0	0	0
inflammation (abscess and mastitis)	7	1	0	1	5

Speed of enhancement finally is assessed most accurately in dynamic studies. Our results with these studies in over 70 preoperative patients are summarized in Figure 7. As shown, the majority of carcinomas enhance fast, whereas most benign lesions, such as fibroadenomas, nonproliferative, and most proliferative dysplasias exhibit slower signal increase after Gd-DTPA. Therefore fast-enhancing carcinomas surrounded by slowly enhancing tissue are best visualized on early scans after Gd-DTPA injection. This is already considered in our standard technique (pages 26–31), but, of course, remains subject to further improvements of equipment and software design. Since, however, some carcinomas (3 of our 24 dynamically examined carcinomas) also exhibit a delayed type of enhancement, delayed enhancement may not be used as a certain reliable criterion for exclusion of malignancy. For this reason and since dynamic studies are only possible in a limited number of slices, we simply estimate speed of enhancement in our routine studies by comparing

Fig. 7

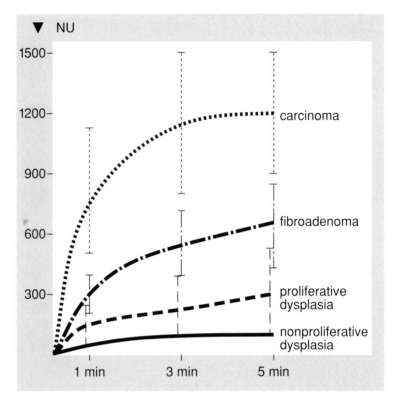

Fig. 7
Speed of enhancement.

The signal increase (mean ± single standard deviation) with time after injection of Gd-DTPA was measured in 76 tissues and lesions in preoperative patients. The biopsy-proven tissues and lesions include 24 carcinomas, 9 fibroadenomas, 10 proliferative dysplasias and 33 nonproliferative dysplasias.

the signal increase of the first and second measurements after Gd-DTPA.

We propose the following simplified guidelines for the interpretation of the MRI information:

– As a tomographic technique, where usually more than 90 images per breast have to be evaluated, MRI is never used alone, but in conjunction with at least mammography and clinical findings.

– The MRI findings are then analyzed and classified as follows:

Group I: no significant enhancement

Group II: focal enhancement

Group III: diffuse enhancement.

No significant enhancement (Group I) excludes malignancy with high reliability, provided the lesion in question was included in the imaging volume and is larger than the slice thickness used. This finding is checked by clinical examination and mammography.

Focal enhancement (Group II) indicates a lesion that necessitates biopsy or, in case of well-circumscribed lesions, at least further work-up, including close correlation of imaging, symptoms, and history.

Diffuse enhancement (Group III) is very uncharacteristic. Even though this finding is usually caused by benign disease, malignancy may be present. Therefore, the final diagnosis should rely on methods other than MRI. In case of questionable or suspicious mammographic or clinical findings, biopsy is usually indicated.

The following sections give a detailed description of the MRI appearance of various breast lesions and tissues. Since MRI should always be used as a supplementary method, the capabilities and limitations of the other methods are summarized first, then MRI features are described.

Based on this background, the potential information added by MRI and its relevance for the various lesions and tissues is discussed.

Normal breast tissue and nonenhancing dysplasias

Normal breast tissue and nonenhancing dysplasias will be treated together, since no exact differentiation is possible based on their MRI appearance.

Histologically normal breast tissue is composed of fat, glandular tissue, and loose and dense connective tissue. Amount and quality of these components vary individually with age, menstrual cycle, and hormonal status (lactation, menopause, or hormone substitution). The term simple dysplasia (dysplasia Grade I according to Prechtel, nonproliferative dysplasia) simply describes a qualitative or quantitative alteration of one or more of these components. Thus, a relative increase of connective tissue is diagnosed as fibrous dysplasia or, if cysts are present, as fibrocystic dysplasia. Increased growth of glandular epithelium, which can be intraductal (solid, adenomatous, or papillomatous) or extraductal (adenotic), should be minimal with simple dysplasia. Simple dysplasia, although abnormal, does not indicate an increased risk of malignancy (6, 9).

Mammographically and clinically the appearance of normal breast tissue is quite variable. Dysplasia is characterized by increased density and nodularity. For both normal and dysplastic tissue, the most important finding is the absence of a solid mass or any sign of malignancy.

For this exclusion, mammography is most reliable in breasts with sufficient interposed fat. Clinical examination is most reliable in soft and small breasts. Thus normal breast tissue or dysplasia can usually be diagnosed based on clinical and mammographic findings.

In some cases, diagnostic problems concerning the exclusion of malignancy remain (see pages 12–16): When normal or dysplastic breast tissue appears quite asymmetric, nodular, or irregular, or when a palpable abnormality exists within mammographically dense areas, malignancy is very difficult to exclude.

Cytology helps increase overall accuracy, especially in case of palpable abnormalities, but is not reliable in case of negative findings.

Sonography may be helpful in some cases, especially if a palpable mass or cyst is present. Its use for exclusion of malignancy is problematic, since it frequently cannot visualize intraductal or intralobular carcinoma and has a reduced reliability for detecting carcinomas smaller than 10 mm.

Contrast-enhanced MRI is proving very interesting in breasts with high amounts of dense or dysplastic tissue, since evaluation of the enhancement behavior may provide significant additional information.

On precontrast T1-weighted MRI images, all described components of normal and dysplastic breast tissue (glandular and connective tissue) except fat display low signal intensity. The signal intensity of fat is intermediate on T1-weighted FLASH images and high on SE images. After the administration of Gd-DTPA the signal intensity of fat remains intermediate or high, respectively, while the signal intensity of the other components remains low.

Fig. 8

Normal breast tissue

Fig. 8
Enhancement of normal breast tissue and non-proliferative dysplasia.

In this diagram, mean and single standard deviation of the signal increase, measured in normalized units (NU), is plotted against time after injection of Gd-DTPA. The arrow indicates the threshold of significance, which is at 500 NU 5 minutes after i.v. administration of Gd-DTPA for FLASH and 0.16 mmol/kg Gd-DTPA (compare Table 3). As shown, the enhancement of nonproliferative dysplasia and normal breast tissue is low and delayed.

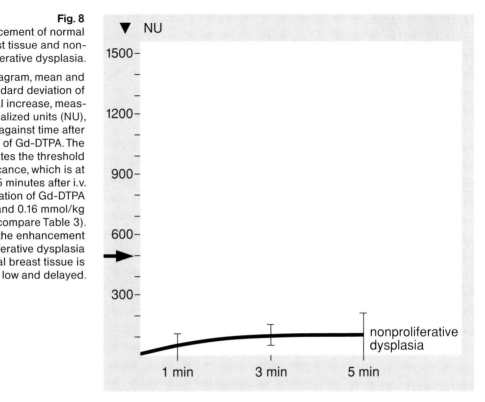

Thus, in general, normal breast tissue and nonproliferative dysplasias do not enhance. If enhancement is present, it is usually low and delayed, i.e. nonsignificant (see Tables 3 and 4 and Figs. 8–11). Since nonsignificant enhancement already excludes malignancy, a dynamic study proving delayed enhancement is, of course, unnecessary for routine examination of this entity.

To avoid any confusion of fat lobules and areas of enhancement, which compared to fat lobules always display low signal intensity on the precontrast scan, all corresponding pre- and postcontrast slices must be exactly compared. In patients with very irregular breast tissue (with many small interposed fat lobules) additional subtraction images of corresponding post- and precontrast slices may be quite helpful.

Figure 9 shows the low and delayed enhancement in a case of asymmetric breast tissue. Figure 10 shows the additional information provided by contrast-enhanced MRI in case of a questionable palpable finding within mammographically dense tissue. In starlike sclerosing adenosis, which mammographically may be quite suspicious, MRI may also help to exclude malignancy, since such strongly fibrosed areas usually do not enhance (Fig. 11).

So far little is known about MRI changes with menstrual cycle, since no intraindividual studies at short intervals have yet been possible.*

According to our own experience, relevant changes of enhancement with the menstrual cycle have not been noticed except in two recent cases (to be published). Therefore and in light of the well-known premenstrual increase of perfusion within normal breast tissue, it should generally be attempted to examine the patients within the first two weeks after menstruation. If this is not possible, a repeat examination after menstruation appears advisable in cases where borderline enhancement has caused any doubts.

Concerning the influence of age, we found that in younger patients normal breast tissue may sometimes tend to enhance diffusely, whereas beyond age 40 very little enhancement is seen in simple dysplasia and normal breast tissue. Sporadically we observed significant and diffuse enhancement after hormone treatment, which then also correlated with a mammographically increased density.

The one lactating breast we examined enhanced strongly and diffusely.

In retrospect, when 91 cases with biopsy-proven normal tissue and nonproliferative dysplasia were analyzed, the vast majority did not enhance. Diffuse enhancement was noted in only four cases (see Table 4). Adenosis, which frequently causes diffuse enhancement and rarely even focal enhancement, is treated with enhancing dysplasias.

This means, on the one hand, that with normal or nonproliferative dysplasia only rarely (4/91) do false positive MRI findings due to significant enhancement occur. On the other hand, no carcinoma has been found without significant enhancement. Our experience concerns over 130 carcinomas in more than 500 MRI examinations. This finding has meanwhile been confirmed by several authors (66, 71, 82, 113).

Therefore, absence of enhancement or very little enhancement reliably excludes the presence of malignancy. Never-

* Gd-DTPA is not yet approved for MRI of the body. Therefore, it has been used on a named patient basis only in diagnostically difficult cases and preoperative patients.

54

theless, to avoid the theoretical risk of missing a small enhancing lesion due to partial volume, we do not recommend MRI for lesions smaller than the slice thickness.

Thus, when MRI is used in diagnostically difficult cases, it should, as always, be used in combination with the other methods. Provided the lesion in question is included on the MRI examination and is larger than the slice thickness applied, we rely on the negative MRI diagnosis in these cases with little or no enhancement and recommend follow-up instead of biopsy.

Fig. 9

Figs. 9a, b
Enhancement behavior of normal breast tissue. In this patient asymmetric breast tissue was detected on the baseline mammogram. Clinically no palpable abnormality and sonographically no cyst or definite hypoechoic area was found.

a) Oblique mammographic view showing the large asymmetric density not present on the contralateral side (arrow).

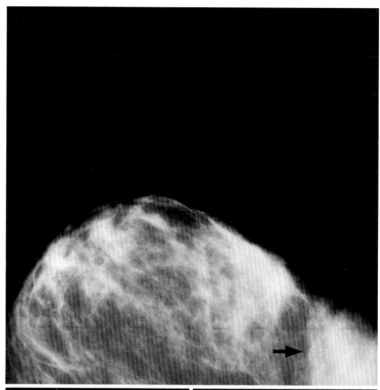

b) On MRI no significant enhancement occurs. Representative scans of the dynamic study (before, 1, 3, and 5 minutes after Gd-DTPA; FLASH 2D: TR = 40 ms, TE = 14 ms, FA = 50°, 0.16 mmol Gd-DTPA/kg). Based on these findings follow-up was recommended instead of biopsy.

Diagnosis: asymmetric breast tissue confirmed by over 3-year follow-up.

from (38a)

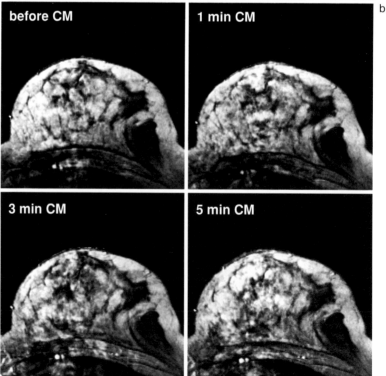

before CM · 1 min CM · 3 min CM · 5 min CM

Fig. 10

Nonenhancing dysplasias

Figs. 10a–d
Patient with a palpable abnormality behind the nipple. Mammographically malignancy could not be excluded for certain because of the dense tissue. Sonographically no definite abnormality was seen, but the study was impaired by shadowing.

a) Mammogram, craniocaudad view.

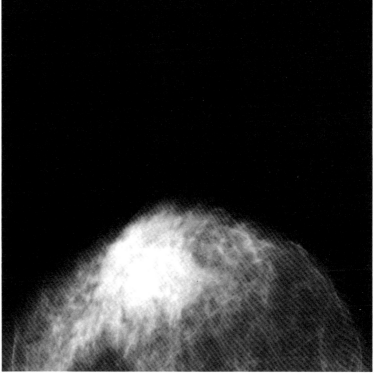

b) Sonogram of this area.

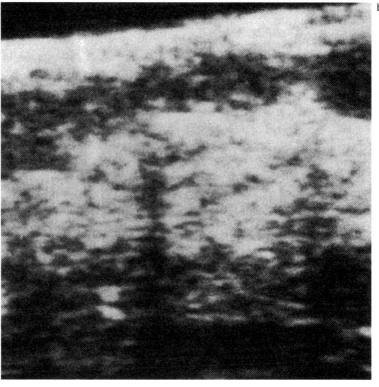

Fig. 10

c) T1-weighted plain MR image (SE: TR = 500 ms, TE = 17 ms) shows dense tissue at the site of the palpable abnormality (arrow).

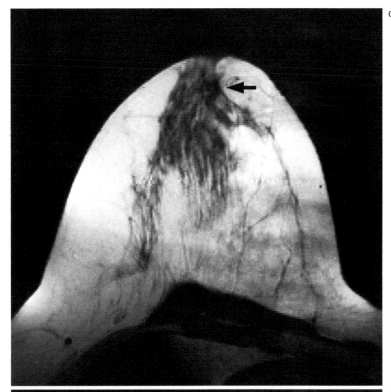

c

d) On the T1-weighted MR image 5 minutes after administration of Gd-DTPA (same slice, same pulse sequence), no enhancement is visible, compatible with benign changes and no sign of malignancy.

Based on these findings follow-up was recommended. Several months later, biopsy was nevertheless performed.

Histology: fibrous dysplasia.

from (57)

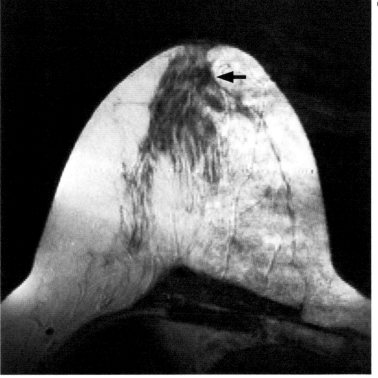

d

Fig. 11   Nonenhancing dysplasias

Figs. 11a–d
Patient with a mammographically detected starlike suspicious density. No palpable
abnormality.

a) On the precontrast scan
the starlike density is identified as well (SE: TR = 400 ms,
TE = 35 ms, 0.35 Tesla).

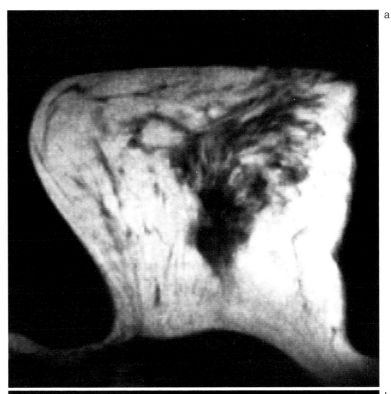

b) After administration of
Gd-DTPA no significant
enhancement is noted or
measured (same slice, same
pulse sequence). The lesion
was therefore considered
benign. Biopsy was nevertheless performed because MRI
experience was still limited at
the time of this study.

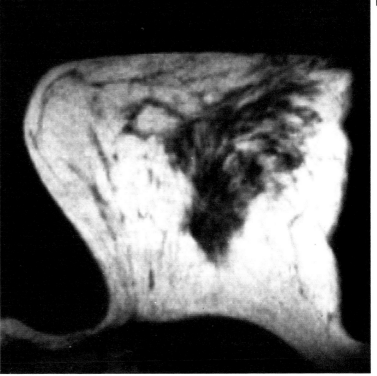

Fig. 11

c) Mammogram shows a lesion highly suspect for malignancy.

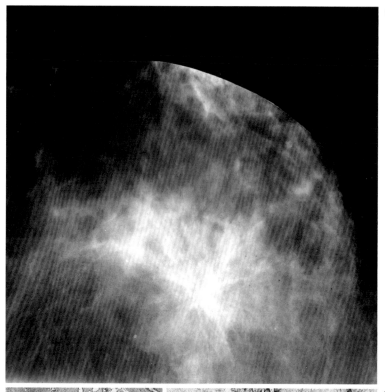

c

d) Histology: a typical star-like scar of sclerosing adenosis (magnification 1:8, inset 1:20).

from (48)

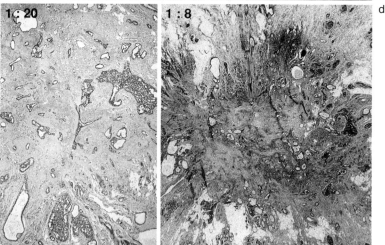

d

Table 3
Dysplasias.
Amount of enhancement measured in 182 dysplasias proven by biopsy of suspicious areas or by correlation with mastectomy specimens. The absolute values and thresholds are valid for our technique and dosage of Gd-DTPA (pages 26–31).

type of dysplasia	no. of cases examined	amount of enhancement		
		2D SE technique 0.35 Tesla	2D SE technique 1.0 Tesla	3D FLASH technique 1.0 Tesla
nonproliferative dysplasia and normal breast tissue	91	120±51 (n=12)	122±80 (n=55)	95±97 (n=43)
moderate proliferative dysplasia and adenosis	76	243±69 (n=15)	370±137 (n=45)	620±293 (n=24)
strong proliferative dysplasia	15	270 (n=1)	526±200 (n=12)	1087±186 (n=4)
threshold of significance		250	200–250	500

Table 4
Dysplasias.
Pattern of enhancement in 182 dysplastic tissues proven by biopsy of suspicious areas or by correlation with mastectomy specimens.

type of dysplasia	no. of cases examined	pattern of enhancement		
		no enhancement	focal enhancement: irregular	diffuse enhancement
nonproliferative dysplasia and normal breast tissue	91	87	0	4
moderate proliferative dysplasia and adenosis	76	9	7	60
strong proliferative dysplasia	15	0	5	10

Enhancing dysplasias

The great majority of enhancing dysplasias correspond histologically to proliferative dysplasias with increased intraductal (papillomatous, solid, or adenomatous) or extraductal (adenotic) growth.

Whereas the association of moderate proliferative dysplasia (dysplasia Grade II according to Prechtel) with an increased risk of malignancy is controversial, high-grade proliferative dysplasia (dysplasia Grade III according to Prechtel) is generally considered a risk factor.

Mammographically the appearance of proliferative dysplasia is similar to that of nonproliferative dysplasia with further increased nodularity and increased density. Compared to nonproliferative dysplasia, the presence of microcalcifications is more frequent. Diagnostic problems may again arise in cases of pronounced mammographic asymmetry, nodularity, or irregularity and in cases with indeterminate mammographic microcalcifications, as well as in those cases with questionable palpable findings in mammographically dense areas.

In these areas sonography is helpful, provided a cyst or even hypoechoic tumor can be identified. But sonography's reliability on exclusion, especially of early malignancy, is limited. Furthermore, areas of proliferation may also appear hypoechoic and thus cause further diagnostic problems.

Cytology is reliable in case of positive findings. Due to an increased number of borderline findings, exclusion of malignancy is more difficult and less reliable than in cases with nonproliferative dysplasia.

On MRI, proliferative dysplasias Grade II and III usually enhance. Since commonly most or all of the breast tissue is affected, this enhancement is largely diffuse and generalized (homogeneous or patchy). Focal enhancement due to focal proliferative dysplasia occurs less frequently (12 of our 91 biopsy-proven cases).

Tables 3 and 4 give an overview of our biopsy-proven dysplasias and their enhancement behavior. As shown, a tendency exists toward stronger and faster enhancement with increasing degree of proliferation (Tables 3 and 4, Figs. 7, 12 and 13). Whereas the vast majority of nonproliferative dysplasias

do not enhance significantly, dysplasias with moderate proliferation most frequently enhance significantly (90%), but the
enhancement is more commonly delayed than fast. Dysplasias with strong proliferation mostly enhance as strongly and
as fast as carcinomas (compare Tables 3, 4 and 7, 8).

The differential diagnosis of enhancing dysplasias either concerns the differentiation of diffusely enhancing lesions or,
rarely, that of focally enhancing lesions:

Since focal enhancement most frequently is caused by
benign or malignant tumors and less frequently by enhancing
dysplasia, biopsy is usually indicated in such cases (see
page 51). False positive MRI diagnoses caused by focal proliferative dysplasia or adenosis – although they are not too frequent – presently seem unavoidable (see Fig. 11).

Diffuse enhancement, in contrast, is most frequently caused
by benign diseases like proliferative dysplasia, secretory
disease, or inflammatory changes, and less frequently by diffusely growing malignancy (pages 104, 130–133 and Tables 7
and 8).

The most important differential diagnosis, the distinction between diffuse proliferative dysplasia and carcinoma, unfortunately is quite difficult and sometimes impossible, due to the
fact that in a small number of carcinomas diffuse and
delayed enhancement may occur. Therefore, only nonsignificant enhancement (in nonproliferative dysplasias and few
proliferative dysplasias) reliably excludes malignancy.
Delayed and diffuse enhancement favors the diagnosis of
proliferative dysplasia, but is not completely reliable for the
exclusion of malignancy. In case of fast and significant diffuse enhancement, exclusion of malignancy is completely
impossible.

To optimize visibility of early-enhancing carcinomas within
those dysplasias with delayed enhancement, it is always
advisable to image the complete breast as early as possible
after the application of Gd-DTPA (see Fig. 26).

In summary, in all cases of diffuse enhancement, very close
correlation with clinical findings and with the other imaging
examinations is necessary. In the evaluation of our routine
cases, we usually recommend further investigation of focally

Fig. 12

Fig. 12
Enhancement behavior of dysplasia with moderate and with strong proliferation.

In this diagram, mean and single standard deviation of the signal increase, measured in NU, is plotted against time after injection of Gd-DTPA. The arrow indicates the threshold of significance, which is at 500 NU 5 minutes after i.v. administration of 0.16 mmol/kg Gd-DTPA for FLASH.

Whereas many dysplasias with moderate proliferation still exhibit a signal increase of less than 500 NU 5 minutes after injection (threshold), most dysplasias with strong proliferation exhibit significant enhancement. The rise of signal intensity is faster in these proliferative dysplasias. Significant overlap exists in the enhancement behavior of the different types of dysplasias.

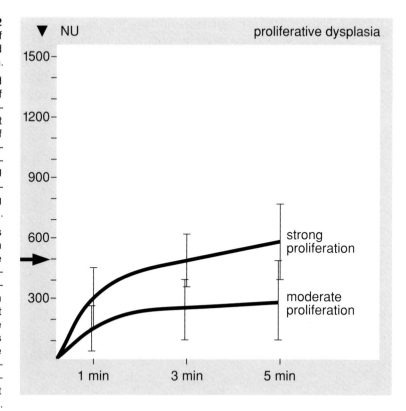

enhancing areas. Mammographic and clinical follow-up is recommended for all patients with diffuse enhancement without suspicious mammographic or palpatory areas. However, if abnormal palpatory or mammographic findings exist, biopsy of the mammographically or clinically suspicious area should be performed. Furthermore, we do not recommend using contrast-enhanced MRI in cases where significant diffuse enhancement should be expected anyway, including cases with known extensive proliferative dysplasia or papillomatosis or with mammographically indeterminate microcalcifications.

Fig. 13   Enhancing dysplasias

Figs. 13a–d
Signal behavior of dysplasias with moderate and with strong proliferation in two different cases.

a) Representative images (before, 1, 3, and 5 minutes after Gd-DTPA) of a dynamic contrast study in a breast with moderate proliferative dysplasia. In addition to the delayed but significantly enhancing proliferative dysplasia (arrowheads), a small fast-enhancing fibro-adenoma is imaged (arrow); it is best distinguished from the surrounding tissue on the early scans after contrast medium.

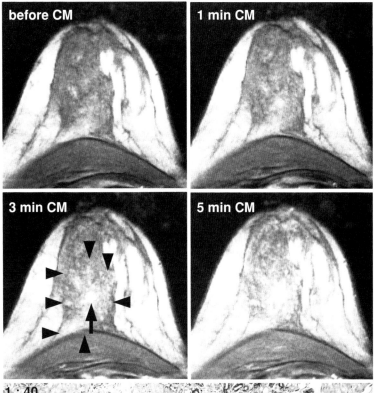

b) Histology: a small fibro-adenoma is shown centrally (arrowheads), surrounded by slight proliferative dysplasia (magnification 1 : 40).

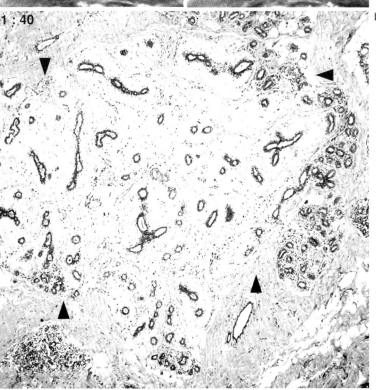

Fig. 13

c) The images before, 1, 3, and 5 minutes after Gd-DTPA demonstrate faster and stronger enhancement in dysplasia with strong proliferation.

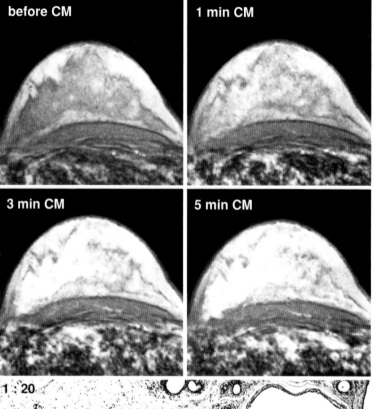

d) Histology: dysplasia with strong partially excessive papillary proliferation (magnification 1:20).

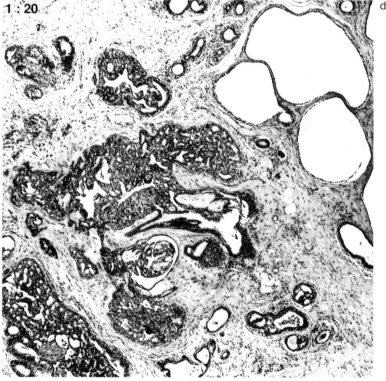

Fig. 14

Enhancing dysplasias

Figs. 14a–e
Patient with a mammographically dense breast with diffuse microcalcifications and a palpable indeterminate thickening of the upper outer quadrant.

a) Craniocaudad mammogram.

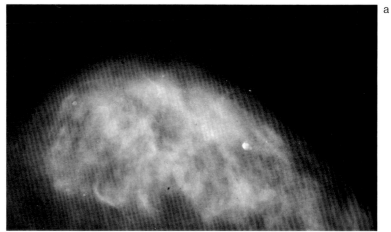

b) Mediolateral mammogram.

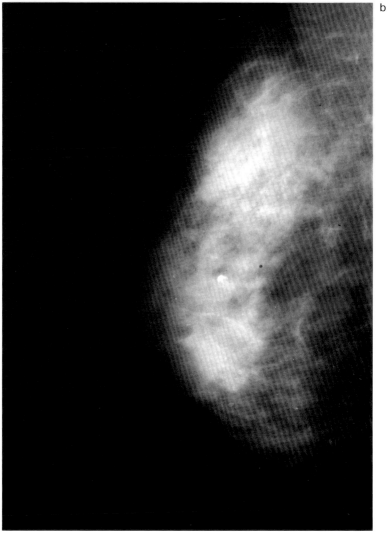

Fig. 14

c) Precontrast MR image (FLASH 3D: TR = 40 ms, TE = 14 ms, FA = 50°).

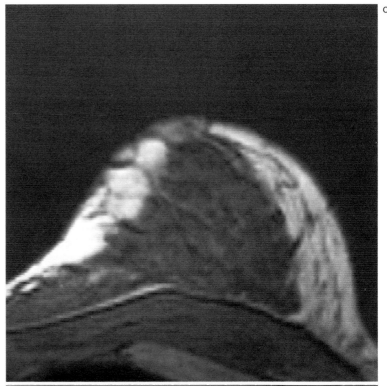

c

d) Postcontrast MR image (same slice, same pulse sequence). Because of both the palpable abnormality and the significant focal enhancement within the same area (arrows), biopsy was recommended.

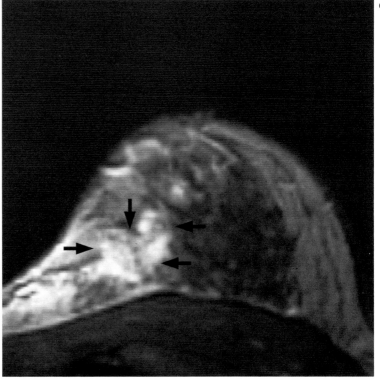

d

Fig. 14   Enhancing dysplasias

e) Histology: dysplasia with extensive adenosis (magnification 1:20, inset 1:50).

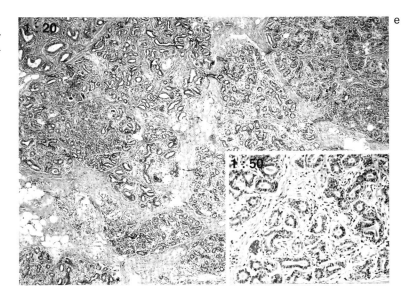

Cysts

Cysts, which are a frequent and harmless finding, are usually related to some kind of dysplasia. Since they can be treated by puncture or pneumocystography, their recognition and correct differentiation from other masses is important to avoid unnecessary biopsy.

On mammography, cysts may be invisible when hidden by dense breast tissue, or they may assume various appearances (round, oval, or polycyclic with more or less well-circumscribed borders with or without halo, sometimes with calcifications in the wall). Thus, the definitive diagnosis of a cyst is rarely possible mammographically. The major information provided by mammography concerns the absence of suspicious microcalcifications or other signs of malignancy in the vicinity of the cyst.

For both detection and diagnosis of cysts, sonography plays a major role. Besides its high sensitivity for even small cysts, ultrasound usually allows good evaluation of the walls, when performed in two planes. However, only when all sonographic criteria of a cyst (absence of internal echoes, good posterior enhancement, compressibility, filling from the periphery when the gain or power is turned up) are fulfilled, can the sonographic diagnosis be considered reliable.

In all other cases, and in those cases where puncture is possible without major problems, aspiration followed by pneumocystography is attempted, since the combination of sonography, pneumocystography, and cytology offers the highest security. Besides detection of intracystic growth (papilloma or papillary carcinoma) and distinction from benign solid tumors, such exact work-up is useful to exclude well-circumscribed malignancies that may be quite hypoechoic, thus mimicking a cyst. This might for example occur in some medullary, or rarely, mucinous carcinomas as well as in some necrotizing carcinomas with quite even internal walls (55, 84, 86, 89).

On MRI, cysts are usually visualized as an additional finding in studies performed for other reasons. However, MRI has also proven helpful in some diagnostically difficult cases where puncture of a small cyst or cystlike lesion is impossible deep in a large breast (Figs. 15 and 16).

On the plain T1-weighted MRI images, cysts usually assume the same or lower signal intensity than the surrounding dysplastic or glandular tissue, depending on their protein contents. In case of sanguinolent contents (see also Fig. 35), however, the cyst may assume high signal intensity. On the usual T1-weighted SE or FLASH sequences great caution is necessary to avoid confusing the sanguinolent cyst with a fat lobule. This problem is, of course, solved when fat-suppressing pulse sequences like CHESS or PEACH can be applied (page 33). After Gd-DTPA, neither the interior nor the wall of the cyst may enhance.

Since all carcinomas enhance, malignancy can reliably be excluded by MRI if no enhancement is seen within the cyst and if very little or no enhancement exists within the wall and surrounding tissue. Only lesions such as a completely hyalinized fibroadenoma (see Fig. 64) or papilloma might assume a similar MRI appearance. Since neither of these lesions requires biopsy, further distinction between such a rare lesion and a cyst is not relevant.

In case of positive enhancement within the lesion, within the wall of the lesion, or in the surrounding tissue, both pattern and speed of enhancement may give further hints as to the nature of the lesion (Fig. 17). However, because of the frequently similar appearance of most of these benign and malignant lesions (papilloma versus small papillary carcinoma, fibroadenoma versus mucinous or medullary carcinoma, abscess versus necrotic carcinoma), in general, biopsy remains necessary in these cases.

Thus, although MRI is usually not necessary for the evaluation of cysts, it may be helpful in some diagnostically difficult cases. In such cases we recommend that MRI be performed either before attempted punctures or at least two months later, since after diagnostic punctures enhancement has to be expected in this area and may thus lead to a false positive diagnosis.

Fig. 15

Figs. 15a–c
Round lesion, which had newly appeared on mammography.
Even though the lesion is relatively well defined, its etiology was not considered certain enough, since sonographically the lesion appeared slightly hypoechoic. Aspiration was not tried because of the deep location within the breast.

a) Mammogram, craniocaudad view.

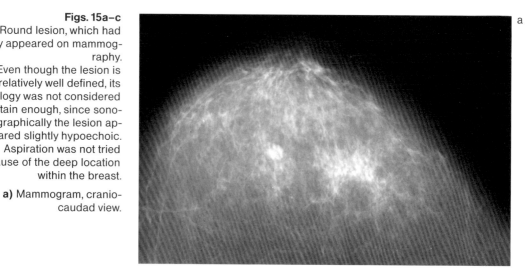

a

Fig. 15

Cysts

b) Precontrast MR image of the lesion (FLASH 3D: TR = 40 ms, TE = 14 ms, FA = 50°).

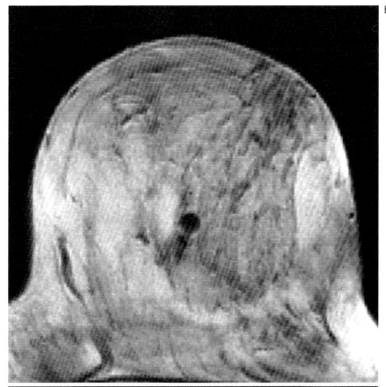

b

c) Postcontrast MR image (same slice, same pulse sequence). The complete absence of enhancement rules out malignancy and strongly suggests a cyst.

Diagnosis: cyst, no change in 1.5-year follow-up.

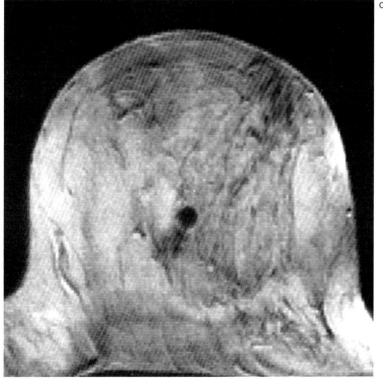

c

Fig. 16

Figs. 16a–c
Another round lesion, detected on a baseline mammogram.

This lesion (arrow) is also relatively well circumscribed. Because of its slightly hypoechoic appearance on sonography, the lesion could not be definitely classified as cystic or solid. Again aspiration was not attempted due to the deep location of the lesion and its small size.

a) Mammogram, mediolateral view.

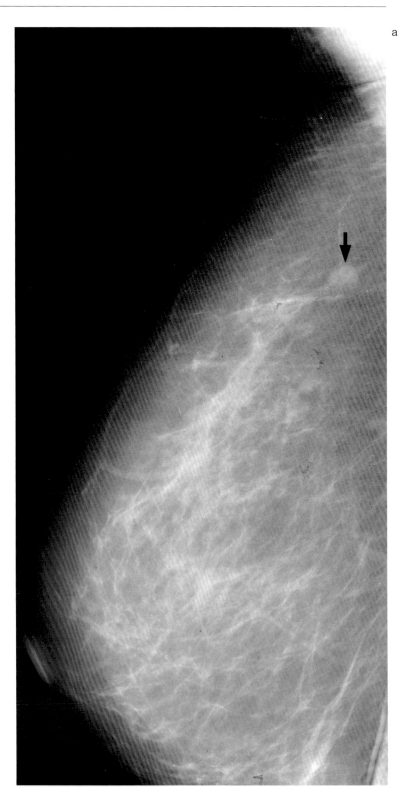

a

Fig. 16   Cysts

b) Precontrast MR image (FLASH 3D: TR = 40 ms, TE = 14 ms, FA = 50°).

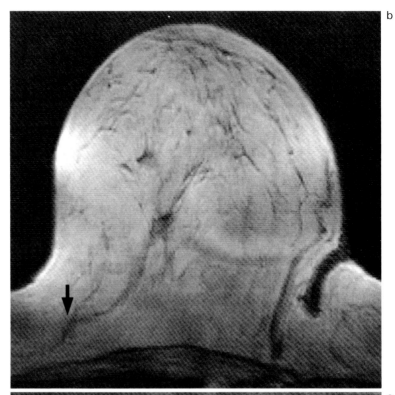

b

c) Postcontrast MR image (same slice, same pulse sequence).
The significant enhancement within the lesion (arrow) indicates a solid lesion. Since a definitive distinction between well-circumscribed malignancy and benign tumors such as fibroadenoma or papilloma is not yet possible by any method, biopsy was performed.

Histology: adenomatous fibroadenoma.

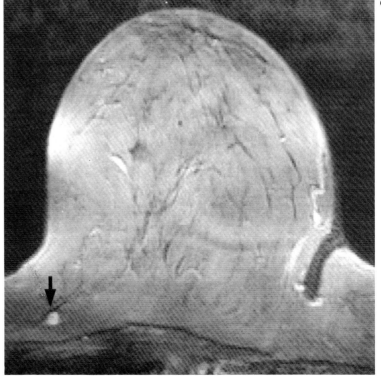

c

Fig. 17

Figs. 17a–d
MRI appearances of cystlike lesions.

a) Nonenhancing round lesions include cysts and completely hyalinized fibroadenomas. Since both are benign, biopsy is not necessary with this appearance.

b) Cystlike lesions with peripheral enhancement may be caused by abscess or necrotizing malignancy. Smooth inner walls, moderate enhancement of the capsule, and diffuse enhancement of the surrounding tissue, extending toward the nipple, favor an abscess (left), whereas irregular inner walls and strong enhancement of these walls favor malignancy (right).
For both treatment and exact diagnosis of these lesions, operation is usually indicated.

c) Enhancing lesions, adhering to the wall, include papilloma or papillary carcinoma. Biopsy is necessary for further classification.

d) Round lesions with more or less homogeneous enhancement include benign and malignant solid tumors such as adenomatous or myxoid fibroadenomas, lymph nodes, papillomas, medullary, mucinous, papillary, or other rare well-circumscribed ductal carcinomas, cystosarcomas, lymphomas, metastases, rare sarcomas, etc. Further distinction is possible only by biopsy (or sometimes by cytology).

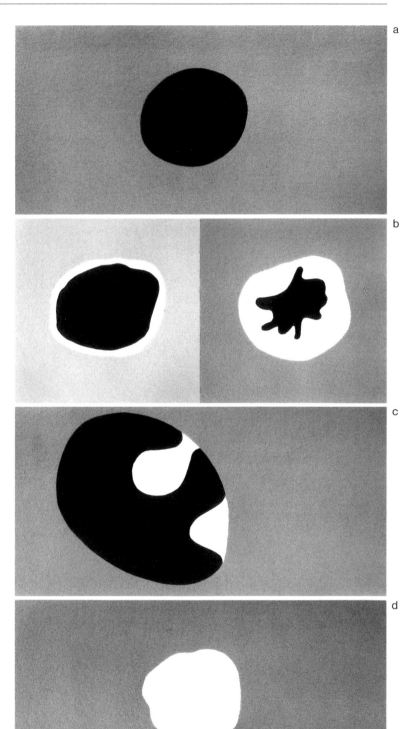

Fibroadenomas

By far the most common benign tumor is the fibroadenoma. Depending on age and hormonal status, various histological appearances exist, such as glandular, myxoid, or fast-growing juvenile fibroadenomas (all containing high amounts of glandular tissue and loose interstitium) and fibrous or sclerosing fibroadenomas (containing predominantly fibrous tissue and sometimes calcifications). Because of both the wide variations in the appearance of fibroadenomas and the sometimes similar appearance of certain malignant lesions, careful analysis is necessary, including various imaging modalities, cytology, and frequently biopsy.

Mammographically the most reliable criterion is the presence of typical coarse calcification, visible however only in about 3% of fibroadenomas (8). Other, more frequent criteria, including round or oval shape, well-circumscribed borders, and even the halo sign favor the diagnosis of fibroadenoma, but are not completely reliable (33, 84, 89, 91, 94, 107).

The same is true for the sonographic appearance, where signs like well-circumscribed borders, regular internal echo texture, and good through-transmission also favor the diagnosis of fibroadenoma, but may be mimicked by certain very well-circumscribed malignancies as well. Furthermore the so-called typical signs are fulfilled only in about two thirds of the fibroadenomas (28, 71).

Lesions that must be considered in the differential diagnosis of fibroadenomas are those well-circumscribed ductal carcinomas that are rich in cells; medullary, mucinous, or papillary carcinomas; cystosarcomas phylloides; sometimes sarcomas; well-circumscribed lymphomas, and finally metastases (8, 60).

Even though cytology can distinguish most of the above-mentioned malignant lesions from a fibroadenoma, it may sometimes have difficulty in diagnosing a fibrous fibroadenoma because of scarcity of material. Furthermore, problems may occur in distinguishing a fibroadenoma from a well-differentiated ductal or lobular carcinoma.

Thus in spite of its benign character, the fibroadenoma frequently necessitates biopsy, since it cannot be distinguished from malignancy. Only in cases with typical history (young patient age, no further growth) and appearance or unequivocal cytology is close follow-up considered.

On MRI fibroadenomas may assume a variable shape, of which oval, well-defined contours are considered typical. The value of this MRI feature is probably equivalent to corresponding mammographic and sonographic features. Therefore, this feature favors the diagnosis of a benign fibroadenoma, but is not completely reliable. The lower resolution of MRI is usually compensated by better contrast, especially within dense breast tissue.

Before administration of Gd-DTPA, fibroadenomas are hypo- or isointense to glandular tissue. After administration of Gd-DTPA, extremely variable enhancement has been encountered, corresponding quite well to the different histologic appearances: Whereas very little or no enhancement occurs in very fibrous fibroadenomas, both speed and amount of enhancement increase with higher amounts of glandular or myxoid components. Thus, most glandular fibroadenomas exhibit intermediate speed of enhancement and intermediate to high amount of enhancement. Very fast and strong enhancement has been encountered in myxoid fibroadenomas. Tables 5 and 6 and Figure 18 show the spectrum of enhancement behavior encountered in fibroadenomas. Figure 19 demonstrates two extremes.

Unfortunately, because of this variable enhancement behavior, MRI does not increase specificity significantly in the diagnosis of fibroadenomas. Only in case of nonsignificant enhancement, which is encountered in very fibrous fibroadenomas, is reliable exclusion of malignancy possible.

In case of delayed but significant enhancement, apart from the frequent fibroadenoma, a well-circumscribed medullary carcinoma, lymphoma, or even a metastasis is possible (Fig. 34). Strong and rapid enhancement is seen in both glandular or myxoid fibroadenomas and in malignancies such as the mucinous carcinomas or cystosarcomas (see Figs. 19, 23, 24, 32).

Although the specificity of MRI in the diagnosis of enhancing fibroadenomas is limited, contrast-enhanced MRI has proven generally more sensitive than the other modalities for detecting fibroadenomas. This fact can be explained by the

		amount of enhancement		
Table 5	type of fibroadenoma	no. of cases examined	2D SE technique 0.35 Tesla	2D SE technique 1.0 Tesla	3D FLASH technique 1.0 Tesla
fibrous	2		220±30 (n=2)	352±128 (n=2)
cellular and mixed type	28	395±94 (n=4)	548±181 (n=20)	1426±313 (n=6)
myxoid	8	585±15 (n=2)	1003±225 (n=5)	2390 (n=1)
all	38	528±150 (n=6)	616±280 (n=27)	1295±641 (n=10)
threshold of significance		250	200–250	500

Table 5
Fibroadenomas. Amount of enhancement measured in 38 biopsy-proven fibroadenomas. The absolute values and thresholds are valid for our technique and our dosage of Gd-DTPA (pages 26–31).

		pattern of enhancement			
type of fibroadenoma	no. of cases examined	no enhancement	focal enhancement: round	focal enhancement: irregular	diffuse enhancement
fibrous	2	2	–	–	–
cellular and mixed type	28	–	20	6	2
myxoid	8	–	7	1	–
all	38	2	27	7	2*

Table 6
Fibroadenomas. Pattern of enhancement in 38 biopsy-proven fibroadenomas.

* similar enhancement of lesion and surrounding tissue

good contrast between the frequently enhancing fibroadenomas and the usually nonenhancing surrounding dense tissue. Fibroadenomas detected by MRI alone were hidden behind dense breast tissue on mammography. Sonographically, small fibroadenomas may be confused with fat lobules or they may be overlooked because their echogenicity is similar to that of the surrounding tissue (86). The higher sensitivity of contrast-enhanced MRI has proven advantageous in symptomatic patients if a questionable abnormality could not be explained by mammography or sonography. Detection of asymptomatic fibroadenomas, however, may pose additional problems because of the presently limited specificity of all imaging modalities (Fig. 20).

Fig. 18

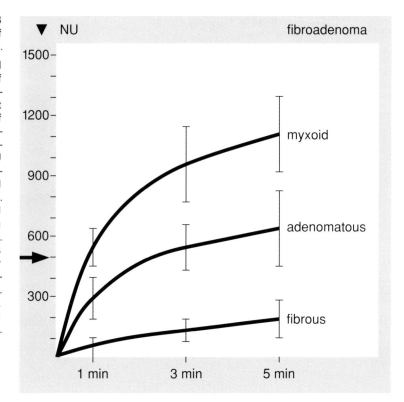

Fig. 18
Enhancement behavior of fibroadenomas.

In this diagram, mean and single standard deviation of the signal increase, measured in NU, is plotted against time after injection of Gd-DTPA. The arrow indicates the threshold of significance, which is at 500 NU 5 minutes after i.v. administration of Gd-DTPA for FLASH and 0.16 mmol/kg Gd-DTPA. As demonstrated, low and slow enhancement was seen in fibrous fibroadenomas. Adenomatous fibroadenomas exhibited variable, mostly significant amount and moderate speed of enhancement. One myxoid fibroadenoma showed fast and very strong enhancement.

In summary, the diagnostic decision between biopsy and follow-up remains difficult and has to consider all data. Since for most fibroadenomas MRI does not increase specificity, we do not consider it a primary method for evaluating well-circumscribed tumors. Only if a fibrous fibroadenoma is suspected (because of hard consistency or less smooth or regular contours, for example) can MRI be advantageous. As explained above, the higher detection rate of fibroadenomas within dense tissue compared to the other imaging modalities has both advantages and disadvantages.

Fig. 19   Fibroadenomas

Figs. 19a–d
Both extremes are shown: Enhancement within a fibrous fibroadenoma (a, b) and enhancement within a myxoid fibroadenoma (c, d).

a) Only slight and delayed enhancement is seen in remaining adenomatous tissue within the fibroadenoma.
The fibrous parts enhance very little.

b) Histology: predominantly fibrous tissue as well as few remaining adenomatous islands (magnification 1:40).

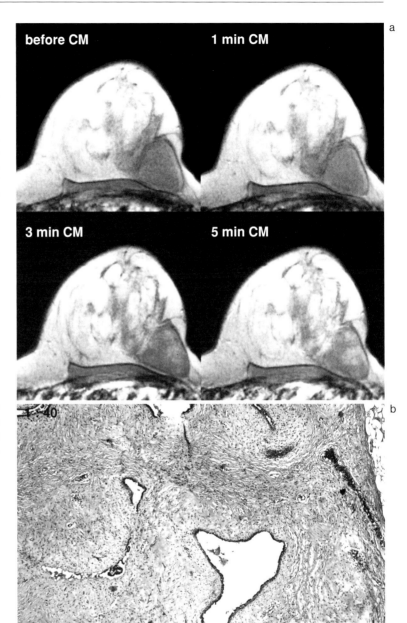

Fig. 19

c) Very strong and fast enhancement is visible in the myxoid fibroadcnoma.

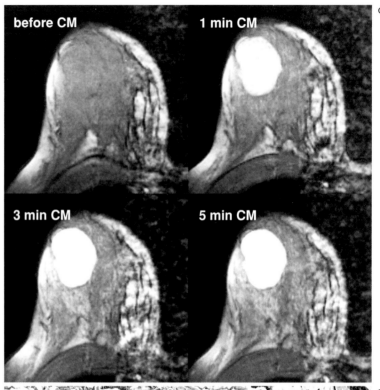

before CM   1 min CM

3 min CM   5 min CM

d) Histology: the myxoid fibroadenoma consists of large amounts of loose interstitium and adenomatous epithelium (magnification 1:40, inset 1:100).

from (53)

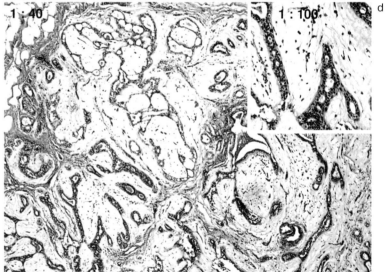

1:40   1:100

Fig. 20

Fibroadenomas

Figs. 20a–d
Fibroadenoma detected by chance.
MRI was performed in this very dense breast because of increased lumpiness in the outer quadrant and the mammographically dense tissue. Sonography had not shown a definite abnormality but was difficult to evaluate because of multiple interposed fat lobules.

a) Mammogram, mediolateral view.

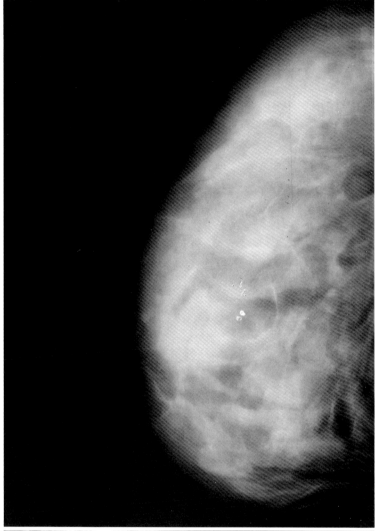

a

b) Sonogram showing hyper- and hypoechoic areas, but no definite abnormality.

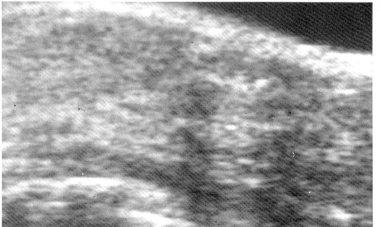

b

Fig. 20

c) Precontrast MR image (FLASH 3D: TR = 40 ms, TE = 14 ms, FA = 50°).

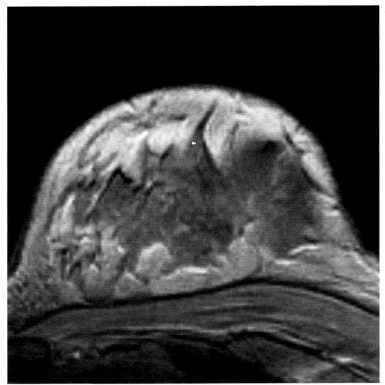

c

d) Postcontrast image (same slice, same pulse sequence) shows a tiny well-circumscribed, strongly enhancing, but not palpable lesion at 12 o'clock deep in the breast.

Due to the well-circumscribed borders and the absence of any symptoms in this area, it was decided to follow the lesion by MRI. Malignancy within the symptomatic outer quadrant was excluded by absence of enhancement.

Diagnosis: probably fibroadenoma, based on 2-year follow-up without change.

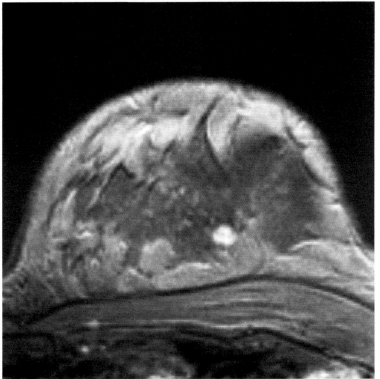

d

Other benign tumors

Lipomas

Lipomas, which consist of fatty tissue supported by fibrous tissue and surrounded by a capsule, are usually well identified by mammography. Therefore, no indication for contrast-enhanced MRI exists. If a lipoma is imaged on an MRI study performed for other reasons, the diagnosis is obvious due to the high signal intensity of fat on the precontrast scans.

Hamartomas

The same applies to hamartomas. They consist of normal breast tissue, usually some fat, and possibly adenomatous or dysplastic changes within this tissue. Mammography usually recognizes the typical capsule and the fatty component of hamartomas without the need for other methods (9, 60).

On MRI, two of four hamartomas which we have examined – usually in studies performed for other reasons – enhanced (probably because of adenomatous changes); the other two did not enhance (comparable to normal or dysplastic tissue) (Fig. 21). If needed, MRI can demonstrate even small fatty components by means of its tomographic imaging.

Papillomas

Papillomas may be detected as mammographic small nodular densities, sometimes with calcifications, or – if hidden within glandular or dense tissue – they may become symptomatic by causing a recurrent cyst or nipple discharge. Papillomatosis, a benign condition and special form of proliferative dysplasia (see page 62), is characterized by the presence of numerous tiny papillomas. Although initially a benign tumor, larger papillomas especially may turn malignant (8, 121). Therefore, and to exclude other malignancies, further investigation of the above-mentioned symptoms or signs is always indicated.

In case of nipple discharge, galactography is the method of choice after mammography has excluded obvious malignancy. Galactography optimally shows intraluminal defects within the ducts.

In case of a recurrent cyst, ultrasound or pneumocystography is usually helpful to demonstrate intracystic growth. If these methods detect an abnormality compatible with a papilloma, biopsy usually is necessary for further differentiation and exclusion of malignancy.

On MRI all papillomas display low signal intensity on the pre-contrast scan. After administration of Gd–DTPA, so far all biopsy-proven papillomas – except one completely fibrosed papilloma – enhanced significantly (see Fig. 22) and were thus visualized as nodular lesions.

Based on amount, shape or speed of enhancement no distinction can be made between a benign papilloma, a malignant papilloma, another malignancy or a fibroadenoma. Therefore, biopsy is usually necessary for further differentiation (see Fig. 30).

The usually very high sensitivity of MRI with Gd–DTPA for even small enhancing benign tumors is advantageous, but it may be problematic as well, as already mentioned in the case of fibroadenomas (pages 76, 77): MRI can detect and demonstrate a papilloma within dense breast tissue or within the wall of a cyst. This finding is helpful if the lesion is symptomatic and if the other methods are inconclusive. However, the very high sensitivity for all tiny enhancing lesions (including benign tumors) within asymptomatic breasts is problematic due to the limited specificity of all methods. In cases where a tiny nodular asymptomatic lesion is detected by MRI alone, we generally prefer to follow up the benign-appearing lesion instead of recommending too many biopsies (14, 63).

In case of nipple discharge, which may be a symptom of papillomas or papillomatosis, MRI is not recommended, since unspecific generalized enhancement, probably due to accompanying inflammatory reaction, has to be expected anyway, and since malignancy then cannot be excluded.

Fig. 21   Hamartomas

Figs. 21a–f
Hamartoma.

a) Mammographically
obvious hamartoma.

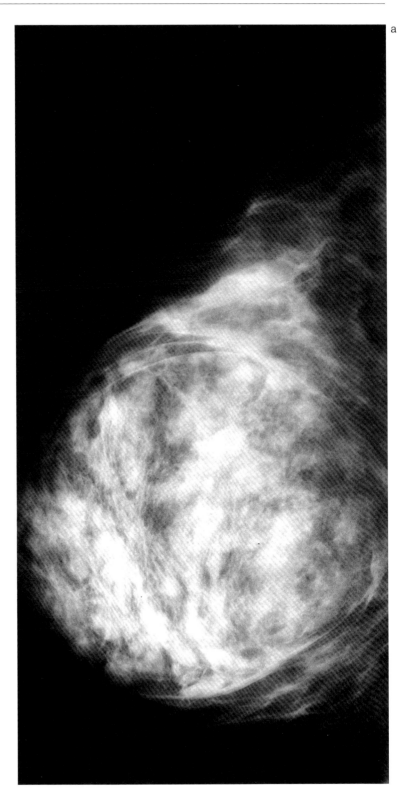

a

Fig. 21

b) Precontrast MR image
(FLASH 3D: TR = 40 ms,
TE = 14 ms, FA = 50°).

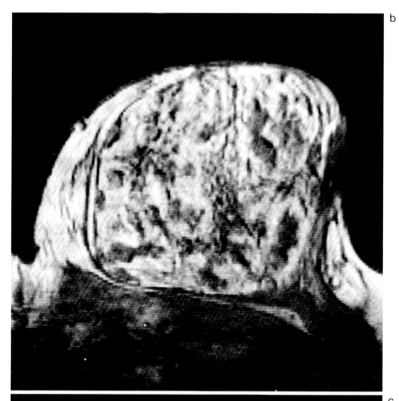

b

c) Postcontrast MR image
(same slice, same pulse
sequence). Significant
patchy enhancement is seen
within the hamartoma,
probably corresponding to
adenomatous tissue. The
diffusely enhancing tissue in
the axillary tail was biopsied
and contained lobular
hyperplasia.

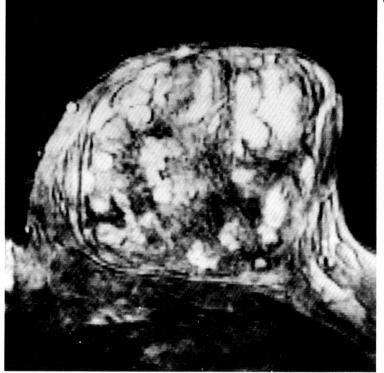

c

Fig. 21   Hamartomas

d) In this patient, mammographically prominent asymmetric tissue (arrows) was
present in one breast only.

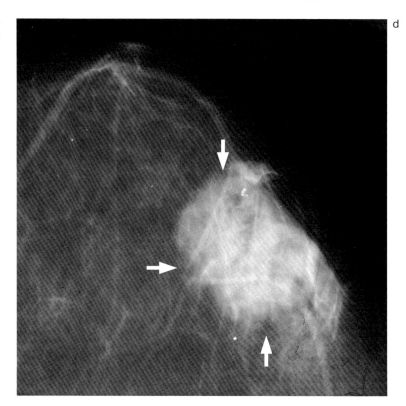

d

Fig. 21

e) Precontrast MR image
(FLASH 3D: TR = 40 ms,
TE = 14 ms, FA = 50°)
shows the dense tissue
(arrows) containing small
islands of fat (arrowheads).
No obvious capsule is identified mammographically
or on MRI.

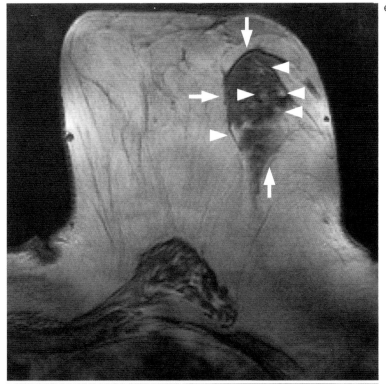

f) Postcontrast MR image
(same slice, same pulse
sequence). The absence of
enhancement excludes
malignancy.

The diagnosis of a hamar-
toma was finally supported
by films from 10 years before,
which proved no change.

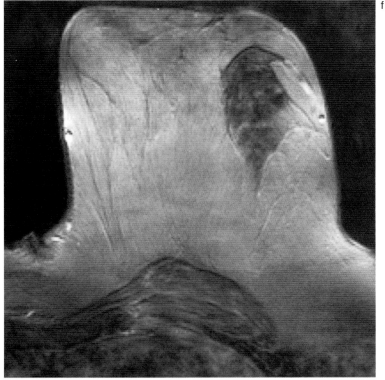

Fig. 22   Papillomas

Figs. 22a–d
Papillomas.
The patient presented after excision of a malignant axillary lymph node, status post subcutaneous mastectomy because of proliferative dysplasia several years ago. No palpable abnormality. Mammography was difficult to evaluate because of scarring, dense tissue, and the implant.

a) Precontrast MR image (FLASH 3D: TR = 40 ms, TE = 14 ms, FA = 50°).

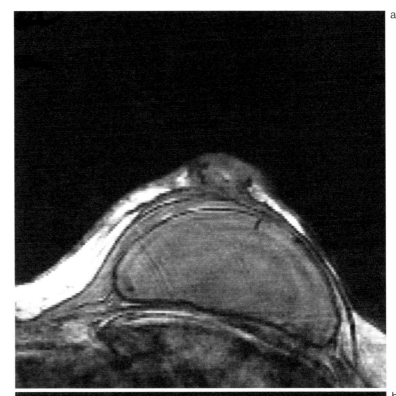

a

b) Postcontrast MR image (same slice, same pulse sequence). The nodular area behind the nipple exhibits strong enhancement (arrows), biopsy recommended.

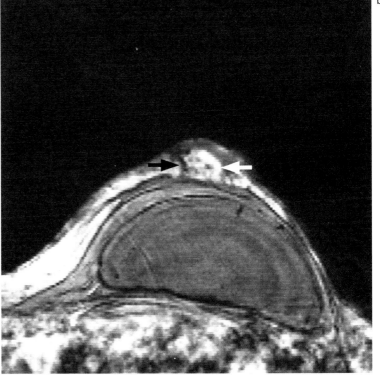

b

Fig. 22

c) Mammogram, cranio-caudad view.

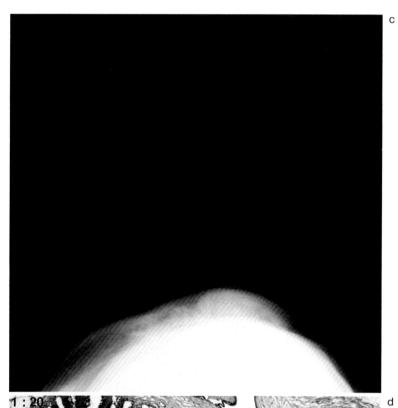

d) Histology: nodular tissue consisting of multiple intra-ductal papillomas (magnification 1:20).

Two years later the primary tumor, a thyroid cancer, was detected.

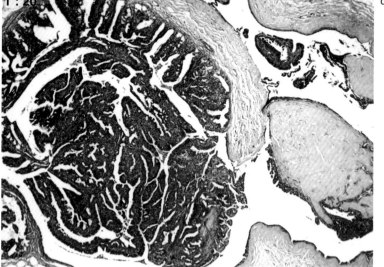

"Cystosarcoma phylloides"

Because of frequent local recurrences (about 30%), "cystosarcoma phylloides" is considered at least a semimalignant tumor. Histologically the term is applied to tumors similar to fibroadenomas, rich with cells, which exhibit an atypical stromatous component with increased rates of mitosis. The malignant cystosarcoma is not common. Histologically malignant changes, if present, may be within the epithelial or mainly within the stromatous component (5, 99). The malignant "cystosarcoma phylloides" metastasizes chiefly by the hematogeneous route (85, 99).

Because of its macroscopic similarity to fibroadenomas rich in cells, clinical, mammographic, or sonographic distinction or recognition appears important, but is – especially in smaller tumors – usually impossible. Clinically, mammographically, and sonographically the cystosarcoma most frequently exhibits benign features, presenting as a well-circumscribed round or lobulated smooth mass. Suspicion is raised when typical sudden, fast growth is reported or when sonographically cystic or hemorrhagic areas are noted within such a smooth, usually larger mass. Osteoid or chondroid metaplasia, another sign of sarcomatous degeneration, may occur, but is rarely seen.

On MRI the one large cystosarcoma we examined exhibited quite inhomogeneous significant and fast enhancement, which corresponded well to the histologic findings of a cellular tumor with necrotic areas. Its appearance thus differed from a giant fibroadenoma of similar size that displayed a lobulated but quite well-organized structure on the T2-weighted image (see Fig. 23).

It appears doubtful whether smaller cystosarcomas (with probably less prominent disorganization or necrotic areas) can be distinguished from the various other enhancing, well-circumscribed tumors. No other reports concerning the appearance of "cystosarcoma phylloides" on contrast-enhanced MRI scans exist in the literature.

Fig. 23

Figs. 23a–i
Cystosarcoma (a–e) and juvenile giant fibroadenoma (f–i).
The cystosarcoma (a–e) exhibits a quite irregular internal structure.

a) Mammographically the cystosarcoma is visible only as a large, fairly well-circumscribed mass (arrows). Coarse calcifications in the surrounding dense breast tissue indicate the presence of several fibroadenomas.

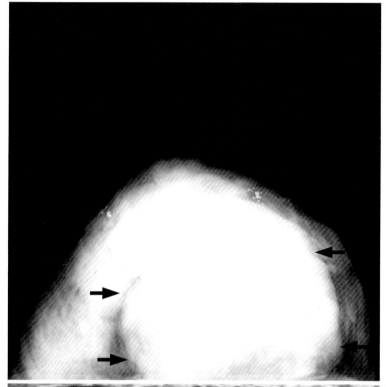

a

b) Sonographically the mass is inhomogeneous and includes cystic spaces at its anterior margin.

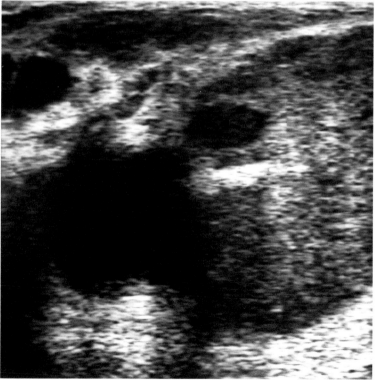

b

Fig. 23

"Cystosarcoma phylloides"

c) On the precontrast MR image the "cystosarcoma phylloides" (arrows) is hypo-intense, fairly well circum-scribed, and sits on the pectoral muscle. FLASH 3D (TR = 40 ms, TE = 14 ms, FA = 50°).

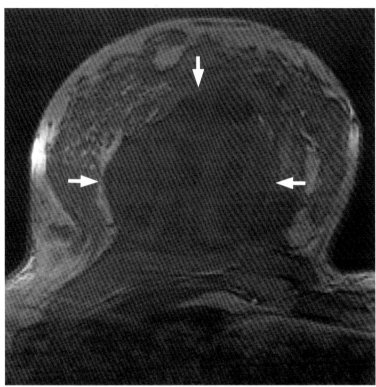

c

d) On the postcontrast MR image (same slice, same pulse sequence) the cysto-sarcoma (arrows) enhances quite inhomogeneously, also demonstrating the cystic area at its anterior margin. Furthermore, several histolog-ically proven fibroadenomas (arrowheads) besides the cystosarcoma become visible within the dense surrounding tissue by their enhancement.

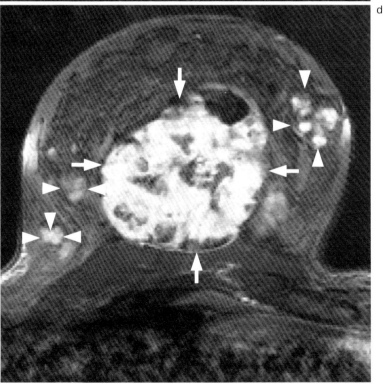

d

Fig. 23

e) This "cystosarcoma phyl-loides" exhibits an inhomoge-neous internal structure: parts look like a giant fibro-adenoma (A). Some periph-eral areas are strikingly lobu-lated (B). Other areas contain significant atypias with sarco-matous appearance within the stroma (C). (Magnifica-tion: A – 1:20, B – 1:20, C – 1:300.)

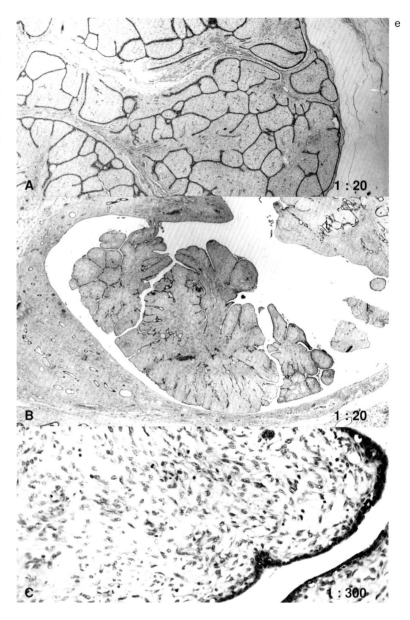

e

Fig. 23

Cystosarcoma and fibroadenoma

Compared to the cystosar-
coma the internal structure of
the giant juvenile fibro-
adenoma (f–i) appears
morphologically more
organized.

f) Mammographically the
juvenile fibroadenoma
appears as a lobulated, well-
circumscribed mass, partially
obscured by the surrounding
tissue.

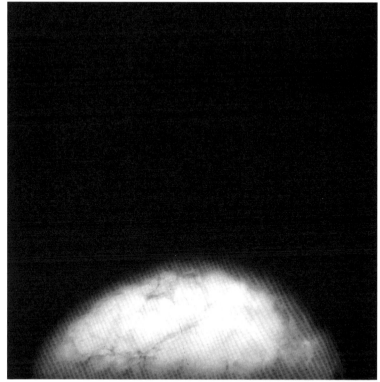

g) Sonography supports this
lobulated appearance.

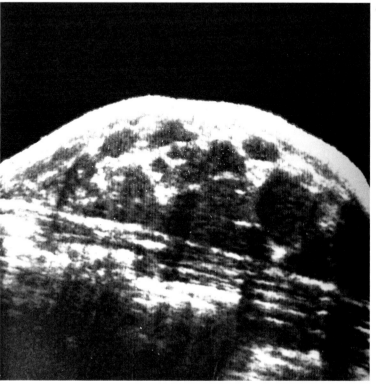

Fig. 23

h) On the T2-weighted MR image (SE: TR = 1.6 s, TE = 70 ms) the "juicy" juvenile fibroadenoma (arrows) can be well distinguished from the surrounding fibrous dysplasia with low signal intensity. Its lobulated structure appears quite well organized (v = vessel). When this study was performed Gd-DTPA was not yet available.

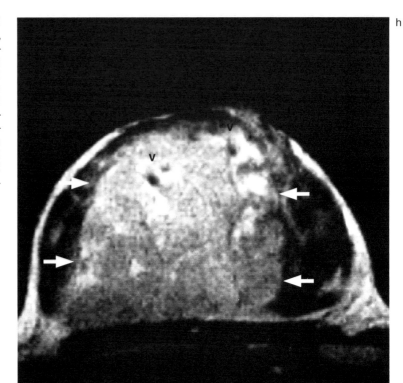

h

i) Histology: homogeneous lobulated architecture of the giant fibroadenoma is shown (magnification 1:40, inset 1:100).

from (51a)

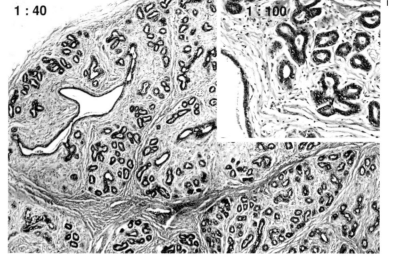

i

Carcinomas

Imaging characteristics of breast carcinomas vary with the numerous histologic types, their morphology and growth pattern (9, 60). For this reason we first give a short overview of the different histologic types and morphologic appearances of breast carcinomas.

Depending on the integrity of the basal membrane, invasive carcinomas are distinguished from noninvasive ones. Prognostically noninvasive carcinomas (especially the intralobular types) need not necessarily become invasive, but they are a high risk indicator. All invasive carcinomas carry a risk of metastatic spread, which increases with size and higher grading.

Noninvasive carcinomas include intralobular carcinomas (lobular carcinoma in situ) and intraductal carcinomas (ductal carcinoma in situ) as well as the papillary carcinoma in situ. Because of their intraluminal growth, they are frequently not apparent to clinical examination and sonography.

Most invasive carcinomas are histologically classified as lobular or ductal according to their origin. Lobular carcinomas consist mainly of monomorphic small cell populations and typically show diffuse growth, often with an "Indian file" pattern, sometimes accompanied by significant fibrosis. The lobular carcinoma is defined by the presence of intralobular neoplastic growth. The vast majority (about 80%) of all breast carcinomas are ductal carcinomas not otherwise specified (NOS). There are great variations in their cytological and histological aspect, from large cell to intermediate cell types, from highly differentiated to undifferentiated forms. The stromatous component also can vary, from low (e.g., medullary type) to very high (e.g., scirrhous type) content of collagenous tissue. Calcifications may or may not be present. The macroscopic growth pattern can be nodular (round or lobulated), irregularly shaped (starlike), or diffuse (within the stroma or within the ducts). Besides these common carcinomas, there are others with a more favorable prognosis, such as mucinous, medullary, or papillary carcinomas, which usually exhibit a nodular growth pattern, and tubular and adenoid-cystic carcinomas. Primary Paget's carcinoma of the nipple, a special variant of an in situ carcinoma, is usually diagnosed clinically, as is inflammatory carcinoma. The latter may originate in any type of carcinoma and exhibits an aggressive lymphatic spread within the skin with an erysipeloid aspect and edema.

The mammographic appearance of carcinomas exhibits wide variations and is determined by histomorphology and growth pattern. Thus, depending on the tumor, different mammographic changes may be encountered. Such changes are called signs of malignancy and include presence of an irregularly shaped or, rarely, smooth mass, microcalcifications, retraction, distorted architecture, increased density, asymmetry, thickened duct, etc. They are used as hints in the search for malignancy. Several or at least one of them are usually – but not necessarily – present in case of malignancy (9, 60, 94).

In general, mammographic accuracy in detecting and diagnosing malignancy depends on both size of the lesion and density of the surrounding tissue. Even though a significant number of small and preinvasive carcinomas are detected by mammography alone, especially small masses in fatty breasts and early carcinomas with microcalcifications in any type of breast, specificity of mammography significantly decreases with the size of the abnormality. This fact leads to significantly worse biopsy rates* of nonpalpable lesions (below 20%) compared to the overall reported biopsy rates (20 to 60%). The wide variation of the reported data further confirms the problems (1, 14, 26, 36, 77, 93, 112). Variation is caused primarily by patient selection (number of symptomatic patients compared to screening population, percentage of young patients with dense breast, and average size of detected malignancies).

As to the sensitivity of mammography, with increasing density of the surrounding tissue nodular, diffusely growing, and preinvasive carcinomas without microcalcifications (about 50% of preinvasive carcinomas) (9) become more difficult to detect. They may even be completely hidden by the dense tissue. Thus, carcinomas within dense tissue are frequently detected at later stages, and a number of preinvasive carcinomas without microcalcifications in dense tissue are detected by chance histologically within biopsy specimens obtained for other reasons (7, 9, 62, 65, 96).

* The biopsy rates indicate the proportion of malignancy among the biopsied lesions.

100

The generally necessary regular correlation with clinical findings can improve only the detectability of palpable lesions within dense breasts.

Cytology may be helpful if it is positive. Thus, highest diagnostic accuracy (especially in dense breasts) has been reported for the so-called triple diagnosis using palpation, mammography, and cytology. In case of negative cytologic findings, however, malignancy cannot be excluded. The value of cytology in diagnosing nonpalpable lesions is an object of controversy (9, 12, 27, 105, 122) (see also page 13).

Sonography can be helpful in the case of questionable palpable abnormalities, if it is positive. Because most carcinomas are hypoechoic, good contrast usually exists, especially within hyperechoic dense breast tissue. However, since some diffusely growing malignancies and above all the prognostically very favorable preinvasive carcinomas may be invisible, sonography cannot be used to exclude malignancy either (34, 74, 86).

Even with the above-discussed state-of-the-art diagnostic possibilities, questions remain to be solved:
– Exclusion of malignancy within dense tissue.
– Differentiation of mammographically detected irregular densities, uncharacteristic increased density, or asymmetry (e.g., caused by malignancy, dysplasia, scarring, or inflammation).
– Differentiation of well-circumscribed masses (see pages 76, 77).
– Classification of mammographic microcalcifications. Even though rodlike or irregular shape, linear arrangement, or significant clustering favor malignancy, a large number of microcalcifications still must be classified as indeterminate.

Summarizing the open questions of present breast diagnostics, both early detection of malignancy within dense breasts and limited specificity in differentiating clinically occult lesions remain significant problems. Increase of specificity appears especially desirable when the radiologist's threshold is further lowered to detect as many early malignancies as possible. Therefore, any additional information is important.

On MRI, all carcinomas display low signal intensity on the precontrast T1-weighted image, as do dysplastic or glandular tissue and benign tumors. After administration of Gd-DTPA all carcinomas enhanced significantly (40, 51, 66, 82). With 3D fast imaging, this enhancement is always visible and measurable. On the postcontrast image, most carcinomas even assume a signal intensity higher than the surrounding fat and are thus quite obvious. With SE imaging the enhancement in carcinomas is always measurable and in general visible when a narrow window setting is chosen. However, on the postcontrast SE image carcinomas usually only assume a signal intensity between those of fat and nonenhancing dysplasia and are therefore not as obvious (see Fig. 3) (59).

In all cases where the amount of enhancement is difficult to assess visually, quantitative evaluation is recommended (see page 31). The treshold for significance of enhancement should be chosen such that at least the double standard deviation of the signal increase in carcinomas is taken into account. For our SE technique it is 200–250 NU* and for our fast imaging technique 500 NU (see Table 1). However, it has to be emphasized that the given thresholds are only valid for our equipment, pulse sequences, normalization and dosages of Gd-DTPA (see pages 26–31). They need to be readjusted with other equipment or technique. Tables 7 and 8 give an overview of amount and pattern of enhancement in 131 biopsy-proven carcinomas examined by us.

In the quantitative evaluation of the amount of enhancement, all malignancies (n = 131) enhance significantly. On SE images all carcinomas enhanced > 280 NU, on FLASH images all carcinomas enhanced > 700 NU. Variations were noted with type and composition (see Tables 7 and 8) (38, 52). Thus, relatively lower enhancement was noted in those small-cell lobular carcinomas with predominant fibrosis and in papillary, medullary, and some intraductal carcinomas. The great majority of carcinomas, including ductal carcinomas and lobular carcinomas without significant fibrosis exhibit intermediate to strong enhancement. Extremely strong enhancement was encountered in the mucinous carcinomas examined.

* The threshold of 200–250 NU is lower than our preliminary estimated threshold of 300 NU. It is now based on the experience of 77 biopsy-proven carcinomas examined by SE technique. This change makes the enhancement of all our carcinomas significant by including even a tiny malignancy smaller than the slice thickness, whose enhancement was initially considered borderline (see Fig. 29).

type of carcinoma	no. of cases examined	amount of enhancement		
		2D SE technique 0.35 Tesla	2D SE technique 1.0 Tesla	3D FLASH technique 1.0 Tesla
ductal	91	481±97 (n=22)	537±147 (n=49)	1182±217 (n=27)
lobular scirrhous	13	368±3 (n=2)	413±98 (n=8)	876±180 (n=4)
lobular nonscirrhous	4		674±68 (n=4)	1533±134 (n=2)
mucinous	4		1093±82 (n=3)	2200 (n=1)
papillary	3		457±150 (n=3)	836±10 (n=2)
medullary	3	315±25 (n=2)	350 (n=1)	
ductal in situ	12	445±105 (n=2)	455±75 (n=8)	910±203 (n=7)
lobular in situ	1		760 (n=1)	
all	131	458±103 (n=28)	526±155 (n=77)	1125±277 (n=43)
threshold of significance		250	200–250	500

type of carcinoma	no. of cases examined	pattern of enhancement		
		focal enhancement: irregular	focal enhancement: round	diffuse enhancement
ductal	91	77	3	11
lobular scirrhous	13	11	–	2
lobular nonscirrhous	4	3	–	1
mucinous	4	2	2	–
papillary	3	2	1	–
medullary	3	1	2	–
ductal in situ	12	5	3	4
lobular in situ	1	–	1	–
all	131	101	12	18

The average enhancement of noninvasive carcinomas was slightly below that of invasive carcinomas, but all enhanced significantly. Variations among them were wide and depended on their type and histologic composition (52).

Although all carcinomas that exhibited microcalcifications on mammography as the only sign of malignancy so far enhanced significantly, we still remain hesitant about using contrast-enhanced MRI (see also Figs. 3, 28, 29, 49) for definitive differentiation of microcalcifications for the following reasons:

– Since microcalcifications are found either within a carcinoma or, frequently, within at least proliferative dysplasia, moderate and sometimes strong enhancement is frequently present in both cases. Thus, too often no further distinction is possible.

– Since microcalcifications may be the only early sign of a tiny intraductal malignancy with a diameter significantly smaller than the slice thickness used, at least the theoretical risk exists that enhancement around such a small area might be overlooked or misinterpreted (for example, as enhancement within a vessel).

As to the enhancement pattern, focal enhancement was seen in about 86% of our carcinomas. In 14%, however, diffuse enhancement was noted. This result was seen either with a diffusely growing carcinoma (7%) or when a focal carcinoma was surrounded by benign tissue with equally strong enhancement (proliferative dysplasia, postradiation or inflammatory changes) (7%).

Evaluation of the speed of enhancement in dynamic studies showed a fast enhancement after the injection of Gd-DTPA in most but not all carcinomas (see Figs. 24 through 27 and 33). In fact 3 out of 24 dynamically examined carcinomas exhibited delayed enhancement. In general, carcinomas with a relatively lower amount of enhancement also exhibited a delayed type of enhancement. Therefore, early imaging directly after the injection of contrast medium certainly improves the visibility of most carcinomas (Fig. 25). However, a delayed but significant signal increase (within 5 to 10 minutes) cannot exclude malignancy (Figs. 27 and 33) (40).

The following examples demonstrate the variations encountered in carcinomas.

Figures 25 and 26 show strong and fast enhancement seen within a usual ductal and a lobular carcinoma. Figure 25 demonstrates the advantage of early imaging after injection of contrast medium. It can be explained by the different speed of enhancement arising from the different vascularity within the carcinoma compared to the surrounding tissue. Figure 26 emphasizes the special advantage of contrast-enhanced MRI within dense tissue: Multifocality in this case was detected by MRI. Figure 27 demonstrates the two extremes: very strong and fast enhancement in a mucinous carcinoma compared to the delayed and lower enhancement within a small-cell lobular carcinoma with significant fibrosis.

Figure 28 shows a small ductal carcinoma that mammographically presented with microcalcifications only (see also Figs. 3, 29, 49).

Figure 29 shows a tiny carcinoma surrounded by equally enhancing proliferative dysplasia. This example emphasizes, that within diffuse enhancement malignancy may always be present (see also Fig. 48).

Finally, Figures 30 through 33 show the enhancement seen in several small or noninvasive carcinomas (see also Figs. 3, 47 and 53 through 71).

Concerning detection and differentiation of malignancy on MRI the following can be stated:

● Absence of enhancement has proven a most specific and reliable finding for the exclusion of malignancy. Since so far all carcinomas enhanced significantly, little or no enhancement reliably excludes malignancy larger than the slice thickness.

● In case of positive enhancement, MRI offers the chance of detecting malignancy not visible with other tests. This is especially true for areas of focal enhancement within dense breast tissue, where the other modalities are less sensitive. However, in all cases of positive enhancement a number of other differential diagnoses besides malignancy must also be considered:

– Irregularly shaped focal enhancement carries the highest probability of malignancy. However, here too, lesions such as focal proliferative dysplasia, focal adenosis, or (in case of status postradiation or surgery) fat necrosis should be considered.

– Focal well-circumscribed enhancement may also be seen in benign tumors such as fibroadenomas or papillomas or in lymph nodes. So far neither configuration nor speed of enhancement appears sufficiently reliable to distinguish these entities from a medullary, mucinous, papillary, or well-circumscribed ductal or noninvasive carcinoma, from metastases, or from rare lesions such as lymphoma, sarcoma, or cystosarcoma.

– Diffuse enhancement is the least specific finding. It is most frequently caused by benign changes and less frequently by malignancy. Such benign changes are in decreasing order of probability: proliferative dysplasia, inflammatory changes, secretory disease, status post radiation or post operation, and, very rarely, normal tissue or nonproliferative dysplasia.

Based on the above considerations, we rely on the negative MRI diagnosis in diagnostically difficult cases, if little or no enhancement is present within the area in question, and if the area in question is larger than the slice thickness used. Therefore, close correlation with all methods, especially with mammography, is always performed. This close correlation is important to exclude lesions smaller than the slice thickness and to provide the clinician with a final diagnosis. This redundant information is especially helpful since about 100 MR images have to be evaluated per breast. In case of suspicious or indeterminate microcalcifications within an area smaller than the slice thickness, biopsy is recommended until the exact accuracy of MRI in such findings can be better assessed.

In cases with irregularly shaped focal enhancement biopsy is usually necessary. If such a lesion is detected and shown by MRI alone, we perform needle-guided biopsy (see pages 33–35).

In cases of well-circumscribed focal enhancement, clinical symptoms, history, patient age, and the findings of the other modalities have to be thoroughly considered for the difficult decision between close follow-up or biopsy (see also pages 76, 77) (14, 33, 84, 89, 91, 94, 107).

Fig. 24

Carcinomas

Fig. 24
Enhancement behavior in different types of carcinoma.

In this diagram, mean and single standard deviation of the signal increase, measured in NU, is plotted against time after injection of Gd-DTPA. The arrow indicates the threshold of significance, which is at 500 NU 5 minutes after i.v. administration of Gd-DTPA for FLASH and 0.16 mmol/kg Gd-DTPA. As shown, the majority of ductal and lobular carcinomas enhance quite fast and strong. Extremely strong and fast enhancement was noted in one mucinous carcinoma examined dynamically, whereas the enhancement in two lobular scirrhous types of carcinoma and in one intraductal carcinoma was more delayed and not as prominent. The overall enhancement after 5 minutes was significant in all types of carcinoma.

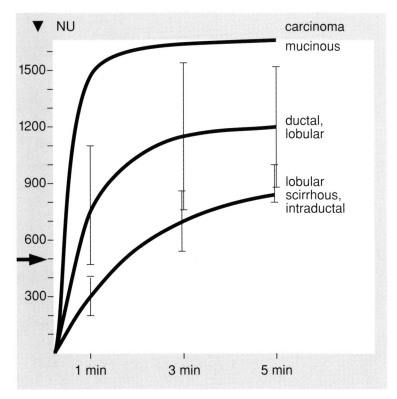

If diffuse or multifocal patchy enhancement is present on MRI, we consider the MRI findings compatible with proliferative dysplasia or inflammation, but we must emphasize that malignancy may be present. We therefore recommend relying on the other diagnostic methods in these cases and biopsy if any otherwise suspicious area exists on mammography or palpation.

Fig. 25

Figs. 25a–d
Enhancement within a usual ductal carcinoma surrounded by proliferative dysplasia.

a) Precontrast SE image of the carcinoma (SE: TR = 500 ms, TE = 28 ms).

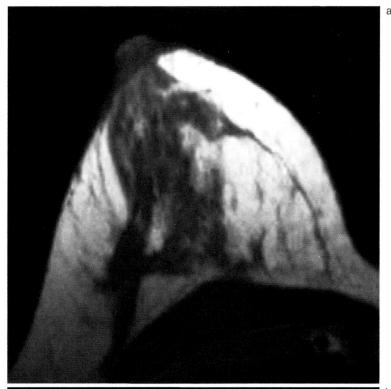

b) Postcontrast SE image of the same slice (same pulse sequence) acquired about 10 minutes post injection. At this time the enhancement in the surrounding tissue is as strong as the enhancement within the carcinoma (arrows). Thus, a distinction between carcinoma and proliferative dysplasia is no longer possible at this time. Compared to FLASH imaging, where enhancement is always visible as a strong signal increase, the enhancement on SE imaging is visible only as a moderate signal increase and the enhancing tissues assume a signal intensity usually lower than that of fat.

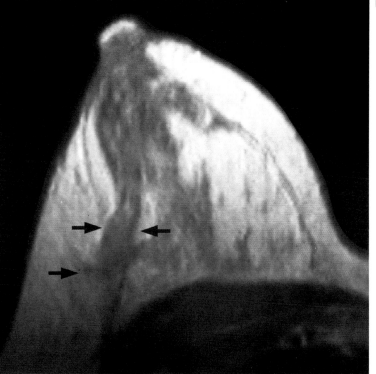

Fig. 25

Carcinomas

c) Representative images of a dynamic MRI contrast study (same patient, same slice as [a] and [b]). These images were acquired before, 1, 3, and 5 minutes after the injection of Gd-DTPA (FLASH 2D: TR = 30 ms, TE = 13 ms, FA = 50°). Strong and fast enhancement is seen within the carcinoma (arrows), whereas the signal intensity within the surrounding dysplasia increases only slowly. Note also the enhancement of the nipple, which has also been encountered in numerous normal breasts and is therefore neither a sign of involvement nor malignancy.

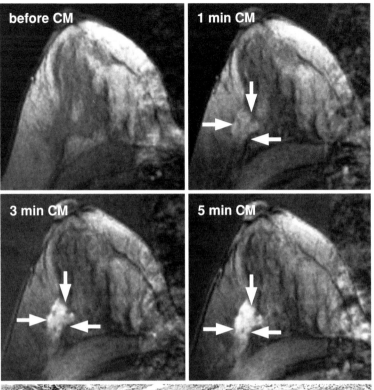

c

d) Histology: invasive ductal carcinoma surrounded by proliferative dysplasia (magnification 1:20).

from (53)

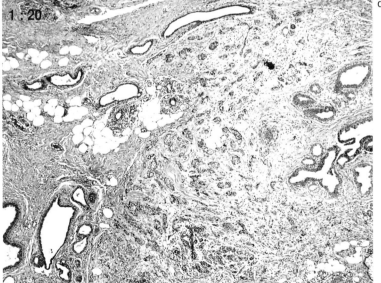

d

Fig. 26

Figs. 26a–j
Multifocal lobular carcinoma in a 33-year-old patient. Since mammography initially had been interpreted as negative in spite of the obvious asymmetry, the patient was referred to MRI. Sonography (performed at the time of MRI) showed one hypoechoic area (c), which was considered highly suspicious on dynamic and SE-MR images as well (d–g). Based on multiple further small areas of significant focal enhancement, multifocal tumor growth was suggested (h, i).

a) Craniocaudad mammogram of the involved breast.

b) Craniocaudad mammogram of the contralateral breast.

c) Ultrasound, showing a suspicious hypoechoic lesion.

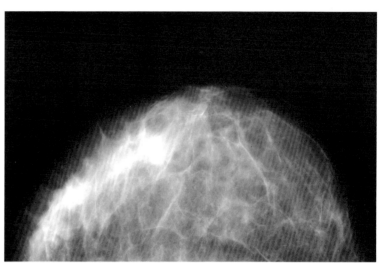

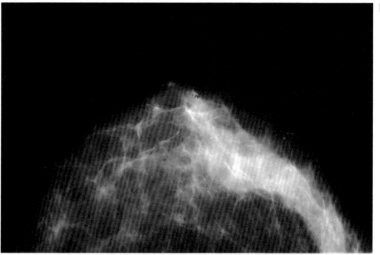

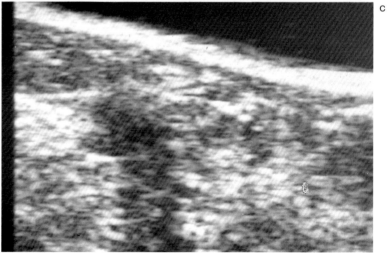

Fig. 26

d, e) Representative images of the dynamic contrast study in the slice of the larger tumor before (d) and 5 minutes after (e) the injection of Gd-DTPA (FLASH 2D: TR = 30 ms, TE = 13 ms, FA = 50°). Strong and fast enhancement is seen within the carcinoma.

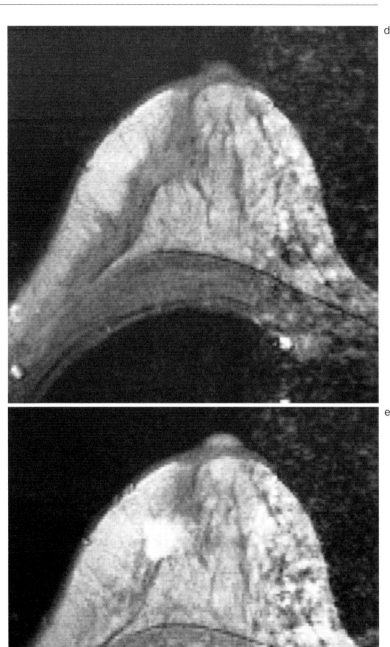

d

e

Fig. 26

f) Precontrast SE image of the same slice (SE: TR = 500 ms, TE = 28 ms).

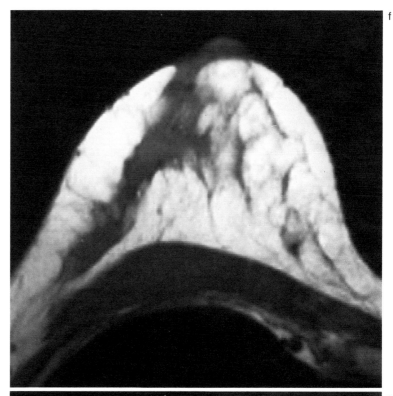

g) The postcontrast SE image of this slice (same pulse sequence as f) was acquired between minute 5 and 10 post injection. As in Figure 25 the signal increase on the SE image is less prominent than on the FLASH image. In this case the carcinoma, however, is well distinguished from the surrounding predominantly fibrous dysplasia, since the latter does not enhance significantly even late after Gd-DTPA.

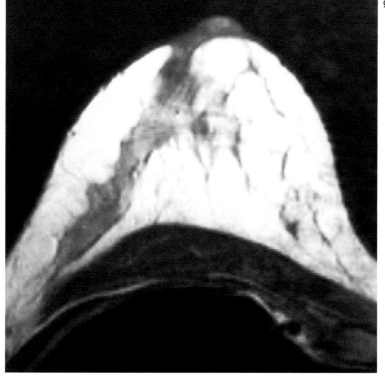

Fig. 26

Carcinomas

h, i) Pre- and postcontrast SE images of another slice demonstrate further small areas with significant enhancement (arrows), suspicious of multifocal malignancy.

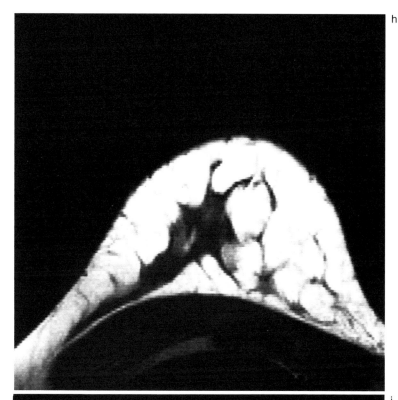

h

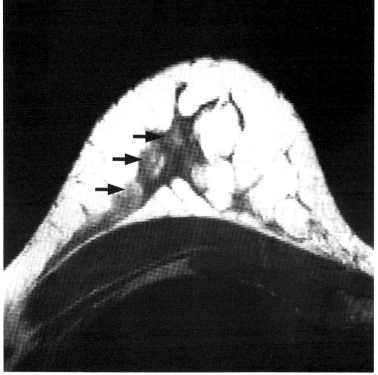

i

Fig. 26

j) Histology: invasive lobular carcinoma with typical "Indian file" pattern. Residual lobuli are visible on the right side (magnification 1:40).

from (58)

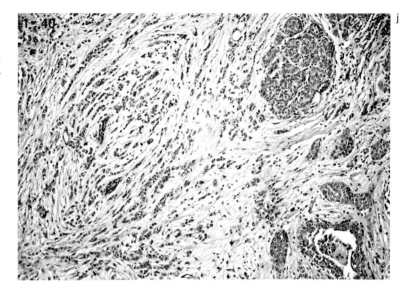

j

Fig. 27   Carcinomas

Figs. 27a–d
Different enhancement behavior of a mucinous carcinoma (a, b) as compared to a predominantly scirrhous carcinoma (c, d).

a) Extremely strong and fast enhancement is visible in this mucinous carcinoma (arrow); representative images of a dynamic contrast study before, 1, 3, and 5 minutes post injection of Gd-DTPA (FLASH 2D: TR = 30 ms, TE = 13 ms, FA = 50°).

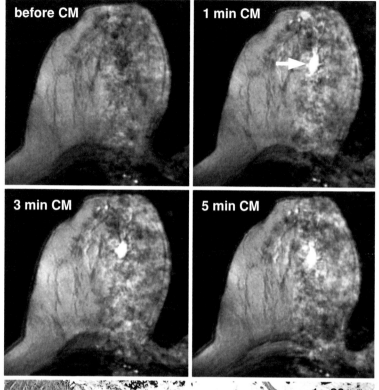

b) Histology: mucous masses with few intermingled epithelial complexes. A relatively well-defined pseudocapsule is visible on the periphery (arrowheads) (magnification 1:20).

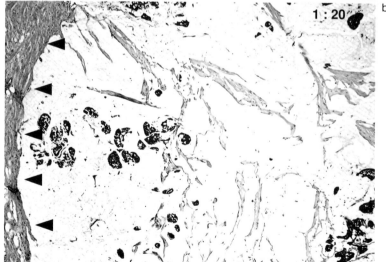

Fig. 27

c) Compared to a), the enhancement within the scirrhous carcinoma (arrows) is only moderate, even though significant. It is also noticeably delayed; representative images of a dynamic contrast study before, 1, 3, and 5 minutes post injection of Gd-DTPA (FLASH 2D: TR = 30 ms, TE = 13 ms, FA = 50°).

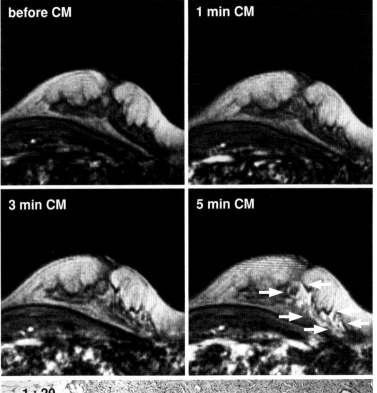

c

d) Histology shows the scirrhous appearance of this lobular carcinoma (magnification 1:20).

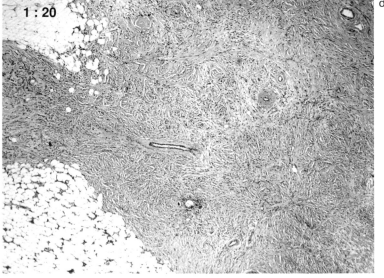

d

Fig. 28

Carcinomas

Figs. 28a–c
Patient with a ductal and intraductal carcinoma, diagnosed mammographically by suspicious microcalcifications.

a) Precontrast FLASH image (one of 32 images of FLASH 3D: TR = 40 ms, TE = 14 ms, FA = 50°)

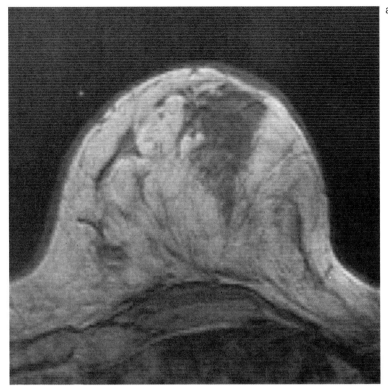

b) Postcontrast image (same slice, same pulse sequence). Significant enhancement is encountered within the involved ducts (arrows), continuing on the neighboring slice. Arrowheads point to some of the enhancing vessels.

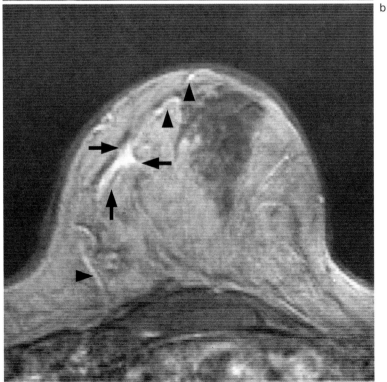

Fig. 28

c) Craniocaudad mammogram showing suspicious microcalcifications with ductal alignment (arrows).

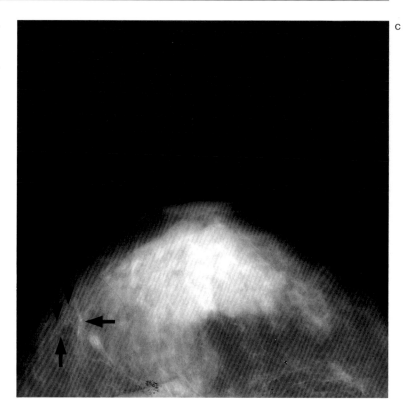

c

Fig. 29   Carcinomas

Figs. 29a–c
Tiny carcinoma within diffusely enhancing tissue.
Mammographically very few
indeterminate microcalcifications are visible within an
area of a questionable palpable abnormality. At the time of
the MRI study, the enhancement was still presumed to
be borderline. Nevertheless,
biopsy was recommended
because of the small size of
the area in question com-
pared to the slice thickness
used. This has proven
correct. Now – based on the
broader experience of over
130 contrast studies of carcinomas – the enhancement
would have been judged as
significant. The example
demonstrates that exact
consideration of all information available helps to avoid
possible mistakes on one
hand. On the other hand it
emphasizes that in the
presence of diffuse enhancement malignancy cannot be
excluded.

a) Mammography showing
few microcalcifications
(arrows, mediolateral view).

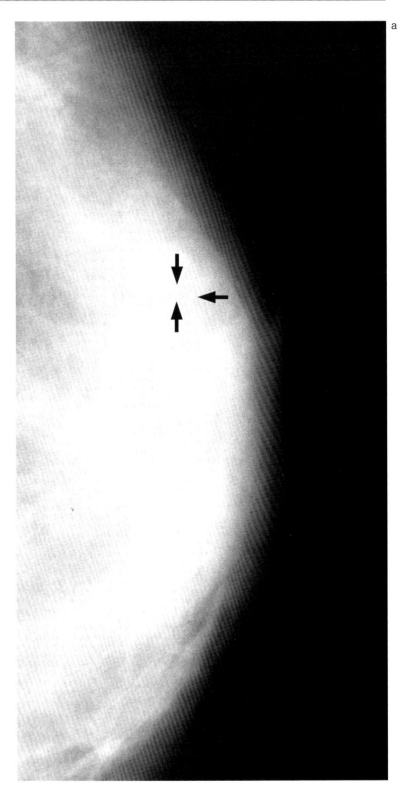

a

Fig. 29

b) Precontrast MR image of the slice in question (SE: TR 500 ms, TE = 17 ms).

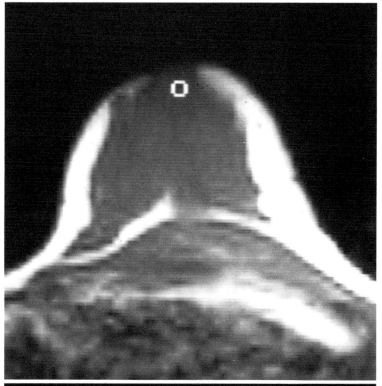

b

c) Postcontrast MR image (same slice, same pulse sequence) shows diffuse enhancement including the area in question (arrows).

Histology: several tiny foci of malignancy were detected within the area in question. Their combined size was still below 5 mm.

from (57)

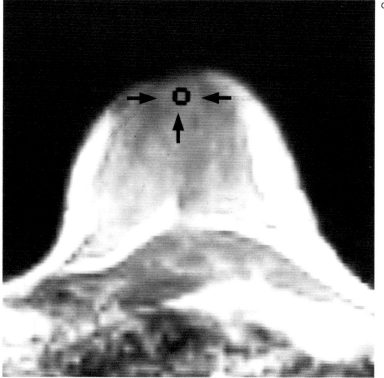

c

Figs. 30a–d
Multifocal papillary carcinoma in situ.
The patient presented with a mammographically suspicious finding and no palpable abnormality.

a) Representative image of the precontrast FLASH 3D study (FLASH: TR = 40 ms, TE = 14 ms, FA = 50°).

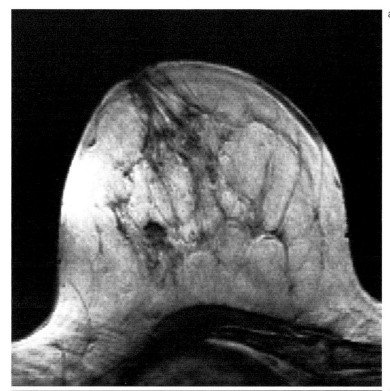

b) The same slice, same pulse sequence, after Gd-DTPA. It exhibits significant enhancement within the mammographically suspicious lesion (arrows). Furthermore numerous other enhancing nodules (arrowheads) were noted in this and neighboring slices (see d).

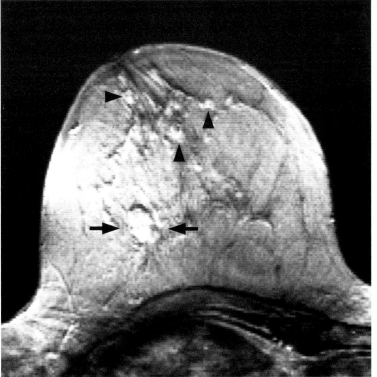

Fig. 30

c) Neighboring slice, same pulse sequence after Gd-DTPA. Several more enhancing nodules of different size can be seen (arrowheads). Based on these findings, multifocal growth was suspected. Differential diagnosis: papillomatosis.

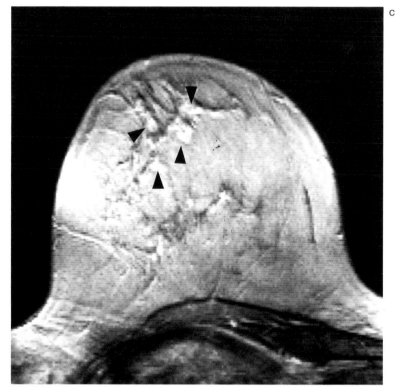

c

d) Mammographically nodular breast tissue is seen, including some coarse calcifications. Only the larger lesion laterally (arrow) had grown on follow-up examinations and was therefore considered suspicious.

Histology: multifocal papillary in situ carcinoma as well as several small benign papillomas.

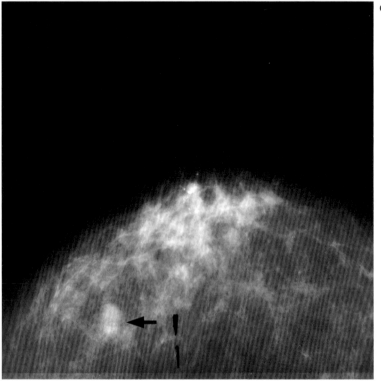

d

Fig. 31   Carcinomas

Figs. 31a–e
Small lobular carcinoma
in situ at 12 o'clock.

a) Mammogram, mediolateral
view.

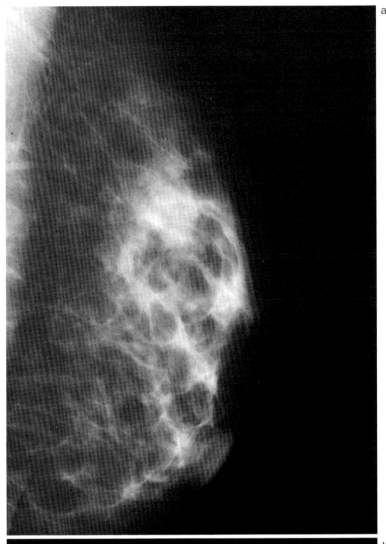

a

b) Mammogram, craniocaudad view. Dense, somewhat
irregular tissue is visible in
the upper outer quadrant;
however, there is no distinct
abnormality corresponding to
the palpable finding at
12 o'clock.

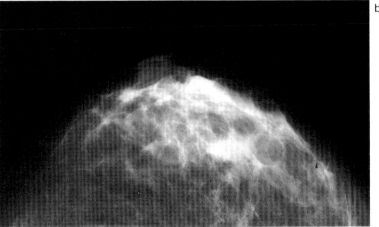

b

Fig. 31

c) Precontrast transverse MR image in the area of the palpable finding (SE: TR = 500 ms, TE = 17 ms). (F = fat lobule)

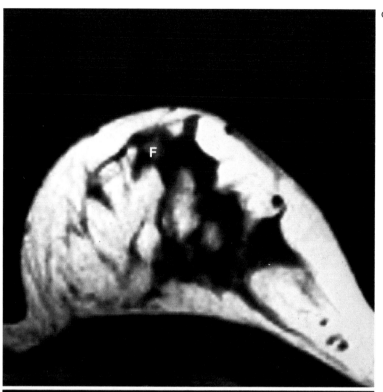

c

d) Postcontrast MR image (same slice, same pulse sequence). A tiny, strongly enhancing suspicious lesion is seen. On this SE pulse sequence the lesion (arrows) assumes a signal intensity similar to that of fat. The fat lobule beside the lesion can be distinguished from an enhancing lesion since it displays high signal intensity already on the precontrast image (F = fat lobule).

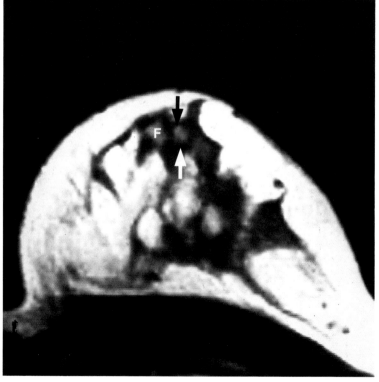

d

Fig. 31

Carcinomas

e) Subtraction image, which results when image c) is subtracted from image d), shows strong enhancement within the suspicious lesion (arrow) and within the vessels (arrowheads). Moderate enhancement is visible within the surrounding proliferative dysplasia.

Histology: small in situ carcinoma.

from (51)

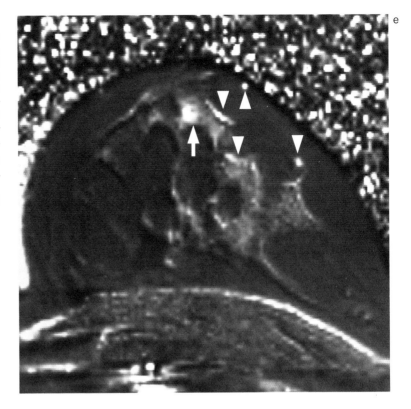

e

Fig. 32

Figs. 32a–d
6 mm mucinous carcinoma in the upper inner quadrant. In this patient with no palpable abnormality, a small nodular lesion, suspected to be in the upper outer quadrant, had been detected on an outside mammogram. However, since among the multiple available views, the lesion was visible only on the mediolateral film, an MRI study was performed.

a) Precontrast MR image (FLASH 3D: TR = 40 ms, TE = 14 ms, FA = 50°) shows the lesion to be in the upper inner quadrant.

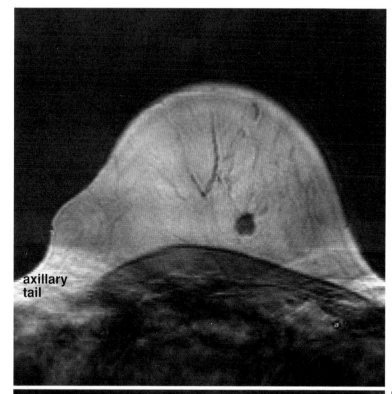

axillary
tail

b) After Gd-DTPA injection, the lesion enhances strongly. As with mammography, with MRI a reliable distinction between malignancy and myxoid fibroadenoma is not possible.

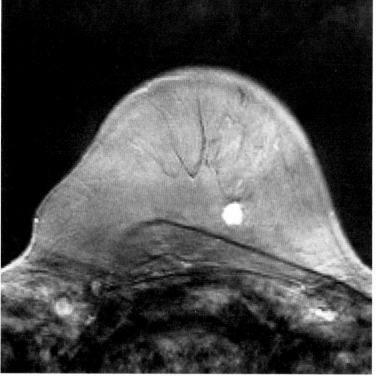

Fig. 32

Carcinomas

c) Mammogram, mediolateral view, showing the lesion close to the chest wall.

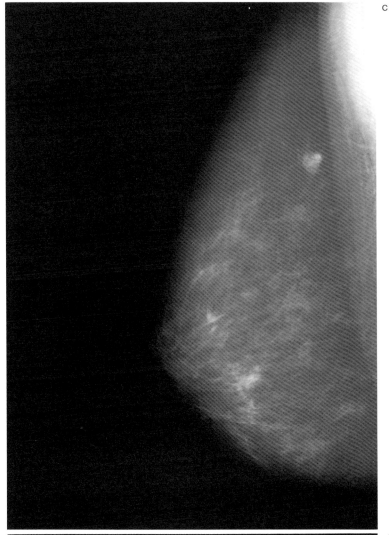

d) Finally, based on the result of the MRI study the lesion could be demonstrated on another medially angled mammographic cranio-caudad view, where the breast was strongly pulled away from the chest wall.

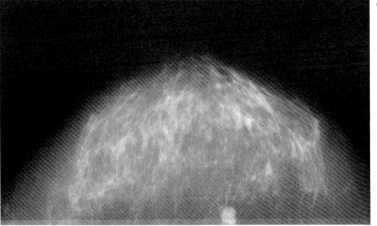

Fig. 33

Figs. 33a–c
Small papillary carcinoma.
The patient presented with a
small palpable benign-
appearing nodule at
9 o'clock medially. Because
of the mammographically
dense tissue obscuring the
area of this uncertain palpable finding, MRI was
performed.

a) Craniocaudad mammogram.

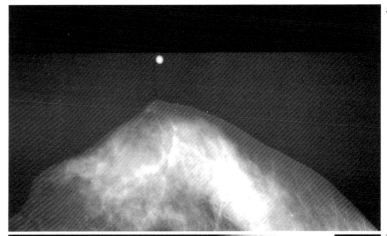

b) Mediolateral mammogram.

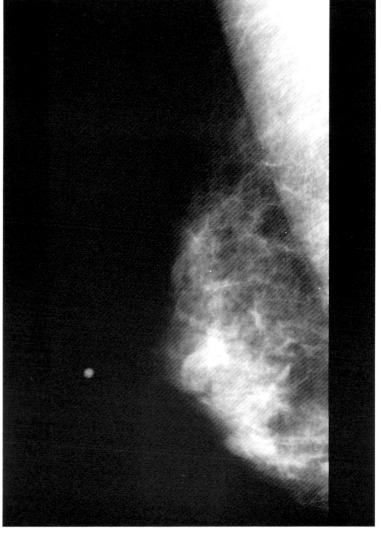

Fig. 33

Carcinomas

c) Representative images of a dynamic MRI study of the area in question (FLASH 2D: TR = 30 ms, TE = 13 ms, FA = 50°) before, 1, 3, and 5 minutes after the injection of Gd-DTPA. Because of significant focal enhancement within the area in question (arrows), biopsy was (correctly) recommended. Note the delayed but significant type of enhancement!

Histology: the lesion proved to consist of two adjacent small foci (< 5 mm) of papillary, predominantly intraductal tumor growth including a tiny area of infiltration.

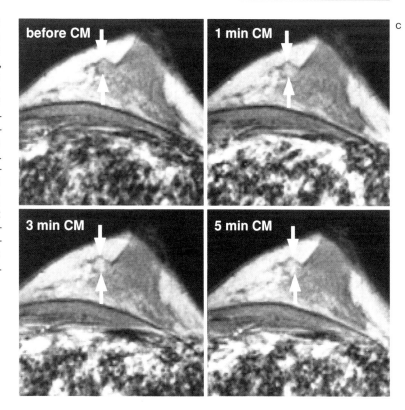

Fig. 34

Other malignancies

Other malignancies of the breast include metastases, lymphoma, or, rarely, sarcoma. As is generally known, all these entities may assume nodular appearances. Lymphoma and, rarely, metastatic spread may also grow diffusely. Therefore, these lesions must be considered in the differential diagnosis of diffuse or nodular enhancement (see pages 77 and 104). Figure 34 shows the MRI appearance of a nodular lymphoma of the breast. So far, however, MRI experience is still very limited. Based on clinical information and other imaging modalities, MRI will probably not play a major role in the workup of these breast diseases, because no significant influence of MRI on the therapeutic consequences can be expected.

Figs. 34a–c
Secondary lymphoma of the breast.
Multiple, fairly well-circumscribed nodules are visualized within the breast tissue. These lymphomatous nodules, which were palpable and mammographically visible as well, enhance significantly.
Histologic proof was obtained of one of them.

a) Histology: a marginal part of one of the lymphomatous nodules is shown (arrows) with some remaining breast tissue in the left corner (magnification 1:40). The inset shows the highly malignant centroblastic lymphoma more closely (magnification 1:600).

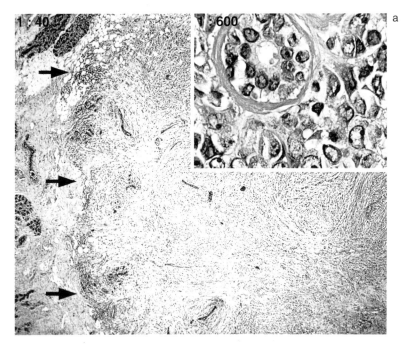

Fig. 34

Lymphoma

b) Representative precontrast image of a 3D FLASH study of the complete breast (FLASH 3D: TR = 40 ms, TE = 14 ms, FA = 50°).

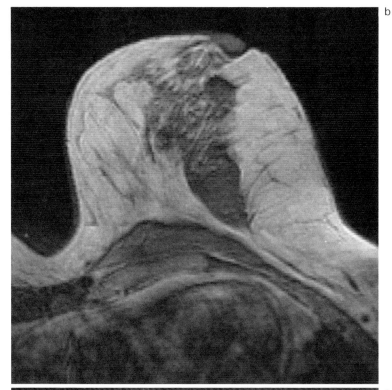

c) Postcontrast MR image of the same slice (same pulse sequence) showing multiple enhancing nodules (arrows).

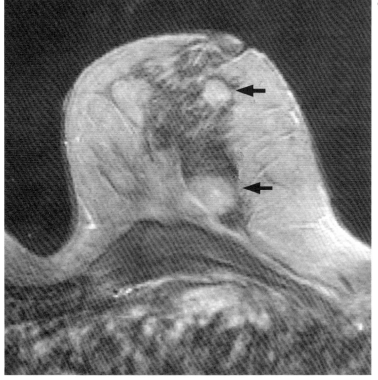

| **Inflammatory changes: mastitis and abscess** | Inflammatory changes of the breast are caused by infection (bacteria, tuberculosis, fungi), by chronic reaction to retained secretion (secretory disease, chemical mastitis) or, rarely, by granulomatous disease (sarcoid, Wegener's granulomatosis) (9, 60). For inflammatory changes after operation or irradiation, see pages 139 and 161–162. |

Depending on the individual changes and their clinical course, diagnostic problems may occur. Besides distinction from other causes of skin thickening like edema and lymphatic obstruction, they chiefly concern distinction from malignancy, since the rare but dangerous inflammatory carcinoma as well as rare lymphomatous or leukemic changes may mimic acute mastitis. Diffusely infiltrating carcinoma can also mimic chronic mastitis. Finally abscess has to be distinguished from necrotizing carcinoma.

In acute mastitis increased density (sometimes more pronounced in the retromamillar area), thickening of the skin and ligaments are seen mammographically. In chronic mastitis, increased density and skin thickening are less pronounced. But suspicious retraction or architectural distortion with irregular densities may occur. The one very specific sign, which must always be excluded, is the presence of typical microcalcification, which may indicate malignancy.

Sonography usually does not further increase specificity in diffuse mastitis, although it can be used to monitor the changes. In case of an abscess, it is useful to demonstrate central liquefication.

On contrast-enhanced MRI, morphology of abscesses is also well demonstrated (see Fig. 35). Signs like smooth well-defined internal wall, strong enhancement of surrounding tissue, and intermediate enhancement of the thickened capsule favor the diagnosis of an abscess versus that of necrotic carcinoma. Since in case of insufficient response to conservative treatment surgery remains necessary anyway, MRI is not recommended.

In case of diffuse acute or chronic mastitis MRI demonstrates the same changes as mammography (thickening of skin and ligaments, architectural distortion, retraction, irregular dense tissue). After the injection of Gd-DTPA, diffuse enhancement is seen. Even though the enhancement in chronic mastitis is usually delayed, we do not consider any MRI criterion certain enough to exclude malignancy (see Fig. 36). Even though only slight enhancement may be expected for most causes of benign skin edema or lymphatic obstruction, present experience is still too limited.

In summary, contrast-enhanced MRI shows the inflammatory changes visible on other modalities. Since it does not in general increase specificity, it is not recommended in the workup of patients with suspected inflammatory changes.

Fig. 35

Figs. 35a, b
Abscess, 2 weeks after surgery.
The abscess (arrows [b]), which probably developed from a hematoma, still contains large amounts of hemoglobin. They are responsible for the high signal intensity of its contents on the precontrast image. After administration of Gd-DTPA little to moderate enhancement is seen within the slightly irregular capsule. Strong enhancement is visible in the tissue surrounding the abscess and extending toward the nipple (arrowheads).

a) Precontrast sagittal MR image (SE: TR = 500 ms, TE = 28 ms).

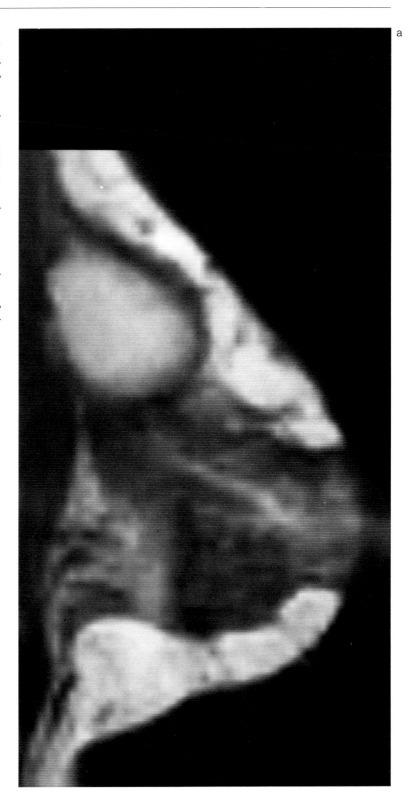

a

Fig. 35

Abscess

b) Postcontrast MR image (same slice, same pulse sequence).

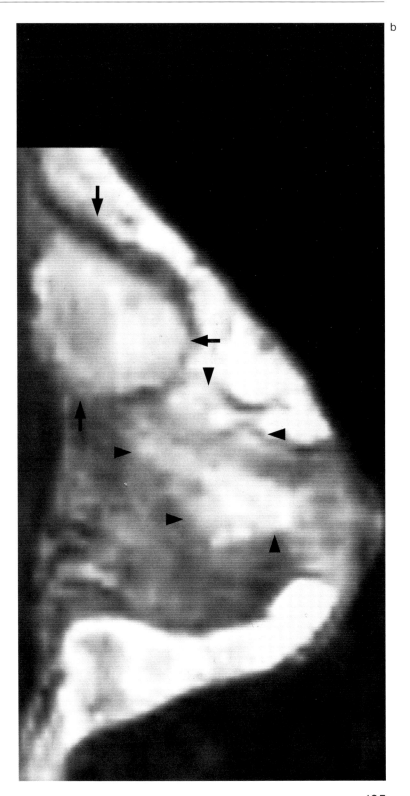

b

Fig. 36

Figs. 36a–d
Diffuse enhancement in a case of subacute mastitis (a, b) versus diffuse enhancement in an inflammatory carcinoma (c, d). Based on the amount or pattern of enhancement a distinction by MRI criteria alone is not possible. In these examples the subacute mastitis exhibited only moderate, the inflammatory carcinoma more obvious skin thickening. Mammography appeared advantageous, since malignancy was strongly suggested by the presence of microcalcifications.

a) Subacute mastitis, representative precontrast SE image.

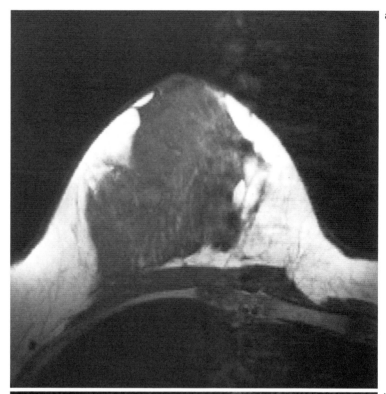

b) Subacute mastitis, postcontrast image of the same slice. Diffuse enhancement of the breast tissue is shown. Only some cysts (arrows) do not enhance.

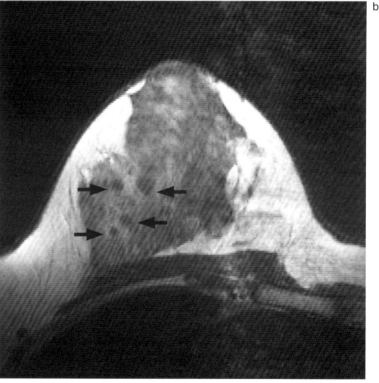

Fig. 36   Mastitis and carcinoma

c) Inflammatory carcinoma, representative precontrast SE image.

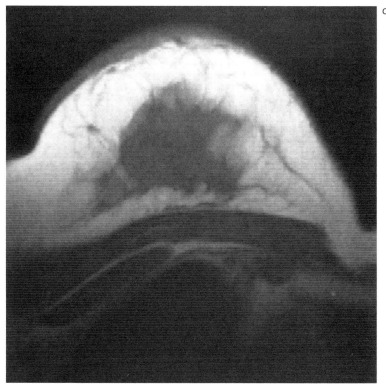

c

d) Inflammatory carcinoma, postcontrast image of the same slice. Diffuse enhancement and skin thickening are encountered.

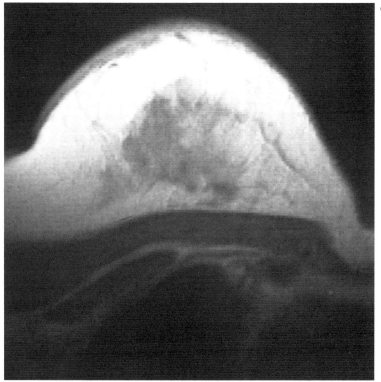

d

Postoperative scarring

Scarring

Based on clinical examination, patient history, mammography, and sometimes sonography, including previous studies, scarring can usually be identified as such. However, in some cases of extensive scarring after multiple surgeries or complicated healing, severe diagnostic problems may arise, especially if previous postoperative studies are unavailable. Both exclusion and demonstration of malignancy may be complicated, since palpatory, mammographic, and sonographic findings in extensive scarring may mimic and/or obscure malignancy (22, 111)

Clinically – depending on extent – increased thickening or retraction of breast tissue and overlying skin may make evaluation difficult.

Mammographically retraction, sometimes starlike, flat and irregular densities or bands (usually without definite central mass), visible on one view only, and ringlike calcifications are considered typical. However, since some malignancies may also be visible on one view only or predominantly and since a few malignancies (especially early ones) may also present with a starlike pattern without definitive central mass (1, 110), these signs are somewhat relative and close correlation with the clinical findings is always necessary. Thus the most reliable mammographic criterion for exclusion of malignancy is decrease or no change of the described findings on follow-up examinations.

Diagnostic problems concern cases where a questionable palpable abnormality is noted within mammographically dense areas in or around the scar (with or without retraction or other distortions). They also concern the interpretation of masslike or irregular mammographic densities, especially if no previous studies are available (which is frequently the case within the first year after surgery) or if the studies are of significantly different technique (different quality, different compression).

Sonography has proven helpful to demonstrate decrease of postoperative changes, especially when performed at regular intervals after surgery by the same sonographer (78). If performed just once, however, differentiation between hypoechoic areas or shadowing caused by scarring and those caused by malignancy is extremely difficult.

age of scarring	no. of cases examined	amount of enhancement		
		2D SE technique 0.35 Tesla	2D SE technique 1.0 Tesla	3D FLASH technique 1.0 Tesla
< 6 months	18	–	275±171 (n=16)	325±206 (n=6)
> 6 months	78	140±40 (n=2)	117±71 (n=42)	138±106 (n=38)

Table 9
Scarring.
Amount of enhancement measured within scarring (with or without silicon implants).

On MRI "young" scarring (< 6 months postoperative) must be distinguished from "old" scarring (> 6 months postoperative). In young scarring very variable enhancement has been encountered within or around the scar (Fig. 37, Table 9). The amount of enhancement ranges from nonsignificant to borderline to significant and depends on the time span since surgery, with remarkable individual variations. The variations can be explained by different inflammatory and reparative response to surgery (Fig. 37). Even though about 3 to 6 months postoperative, this enhancement is usually delayed (compared to the enhancement of most carcinomas) and decreases, exact distinction between scarring and malignancy earlier than 6 months after surgery (< 6 months) is in most cases not yet possible, because significant or borderline enhancement will still be present.

In scarring older than 6 months postoperative little or no enhancement is measured, a finding compatible with completed fibrosis (see Table 9). Therefore excellent distinction between old scarring (independent of its shape and irregularity) and malignancy is usually possible based on the different enhancement behavior on MRI (see Figs. 38 and 39). This feature of contrast-enhanced MRI proved quite helpful in more than two thirds of diagnostically difficult cases with scarring later than 6 months postoperative (50). Table 9 gives an overview of the enhancement measured within scarring.

Finally, it should be mentioned that in several scars independent of their age small signal voids have been noted, especially on fast-imaging scans (see also Figs. 39, 48, 67). They are of no diagnostic importance and their etiology is not yet exactly known, since no histopathologic correlate has yet been detected. These signal voids might be caused by microscopic remnants of glove powder.

Masses that may occur in addition to the already-described inflammatory or fibrous changes within the scar are seroma, hematoma, oil cyst, or fat necrosis (9,60).

Seroma and hematoma in early scarring can usually be diagnosed by sonography and are, of course, also demonstrated by MRI. Oil cyst is usually a quite specific mammographic diagnosis. Therefore, although it can be demonstrated by MRI as well, MRI is usually not necessary for this diagnosis (Fig. 40).

Fresh fat necrosis, however, may cause significant diagnostic problems for all methods (90, 114): Due to their masslike appearance, irregular contours, and sometimes indeterminate microcalcifications, fat necroses may be indistinguishable from malignancy clinically, mammographically, and sonographically. Since on contrast-enhanced MRI, fresh fat necrosis enhances significantly, too, contrast-enhanced MRI cannot distinguish between fat necrosis and malignancy (see Fig. 41).

In summary, because of the very different enhancement of fibrotic changes compared to malignancy, contrast-enhanced MRI offers valuable information in diagnostically difficult cases with scarring older than 6 months postoperative. Based on our experience, we do rely on MRI, if no enhancement is present and the area in question is larger than the slice thickness. The latter is again checked by mammography as well (absence of a tiny focus of microcalcifications).

In case of positive focal enhancement, biopsy usually is necessary for further differentiation between malignancy, other tumors (papilloma, fibroadenoma or, rarely, focal proliferative dysplasia), some inflammatory change, or fresh fat necrosis, which may be the cause of false positive diagnoses. Because of the excellent contrast between scarring and malignancy, MRI here offers the chance to detect early malignancy within distorted scar tissue.

Diffuse enhancement within scarring older than 6 months is quite rare and may be caused by inflammation. In such cases MRI cannot exclude malignancy.

Because of the usually borderline to significant enhancement in scarring earlier than 6 months postoperative, MRI is not recommended at this stage, but could – if needed – tentatively be applied 3 to 6 months postoperative with some uncertainty as to its usefulness.

Scarring with silicon implants

In patients with silicon implants, diagnostic problems may be caused by scarring and by the implant itself (17, 21, 35, 56, 100, 126). As to the problems caused by scarring, we have noted no significant differences between postoperative scarring with or without silicon implants. Therefore, the statements concerning postoperative scarring (see pages 138–141 and Table 9) also apply to scarring around silicon implants. Some specific problems such as inflammatory response to the implant or its contents, increased fibrosis of the capsule, or folding of the implant may occur.

With conventional methods, evaluation of all these changes and exclusion of malignancy is further impaired by the mere presence of the implant, for the following reasons:

– Clinically those parts of the breast tissue close to the chest wall behind the implant usually cannot be assessed adequately.

– Mammographically large parts of the breast tissue not only behind but also around the implant are obscured by the high roentgen density of the implant. Therefore, even when multiple views or xeromammography are used, which may slightly improve the situation by its larger latitude but has other disadvantages (56), mammographic evaluation is quite incomplete.

– Sonography has proven quite helpful as a supplementary tool in these patients, since – with a tomographic technique like that of MRI – it allows assessment of the breast tissue around the implant without superimposition (17). However, problems remain in cases with significant scarring, due to hypoechoic and shadowing scar tissue. Furthermore, exclusion of malignancy < 1 cm and of in situ malignancy is uncertain.

MRI offers the following advantages:

- The complete breast tissue including chest wall behind the implant is visualized (see Figs. 42–44) (50, 56, 106).

– Compared to sonography and clinical examination, MRI provides excellent reproducibility.

– As mentioned on page 139, MRI may allow distinction of malignancy and fibrosis based on their different enhancement behavior.

Therefore, in patients with silicon implants (more than 6 months postoperative) MRI can significantly contribute to early detection of malignancy within distorted scar tissue or behind the implant and to differentiation between scarring and malignancy (Figs. 42 through 45).

In case of inflammatory changes (which occurred later than 6 months postoperative in only two of our patients) or earlier than 6 months postoperative, however, variable, usually diffuse enhancement makes exclusion of malignancy impossible.

In summary, significant additional information may be contributed by contrast-enhanced MRI in patients with silicon implants more than 6 months postoperative. Therefore, MRI promises to become a very important method in evaluating these patients. It should nevertheless be used in conjunction with mammography, which excludes the presence of a tiny focus of microcalcifications within tissue not hidden by the implant. The information provided by MRI gives excellent differentiation between fibrosis and malignancy and tomographic visualization of the complete tissue around the implant. In case of inflammatory changes or within the first 6 months postoperative the value of MRI is doubtful.

Fig. 37

Scarring

Figs. 37a–d
Variable enhancement within
and around the scar in two
different patients 2 months
after surgery.
Whereas in patient A (a, b)
significant enhancement is
visible in parts of the scar
only, in patient B (c, d) significant enhancement is seen
within the scar and within a
larger area of surrounding
tissue.

a) Patient A, precontrast scan
through the scar (slice of a
FLASH 3D study: TR = 40 ms,
TE = 14 ms, FA = 50°).

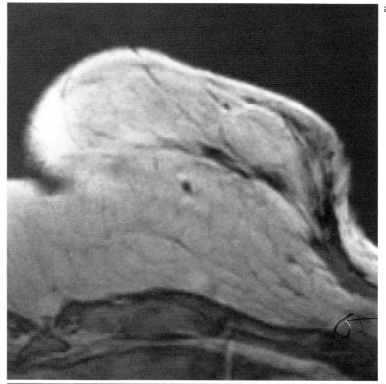

b) Patient A, postcontrast
image (same slice, same
pulse sequence).

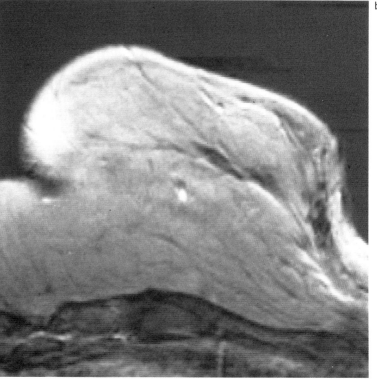

Fig. 37

c) Patient B, precontrast scan at the level of the scar (SE: TR = 500 ms, TE = 30 ms).

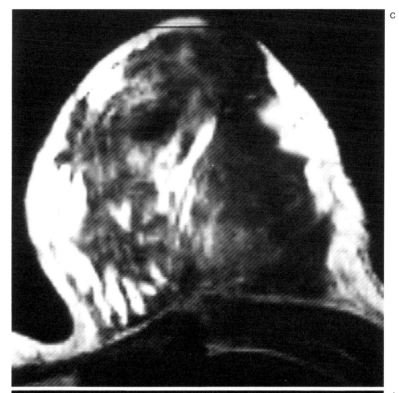

c

d) Patient B, postcontrast scan (same slice, same pulse sequence). Significant enhancement is seen within a larger area (arrows) around the scar.

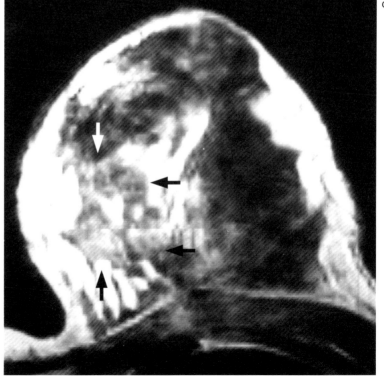

d

Fig. 38

Scarring

Figs. 38a–d
Scarring above 6 months
postoperative.
In this patient, a suspicious
masslike increased density
was noted in the prepectoral
area on the first postoperative mammogram 7 months
after surgery. MRI was performed to exclude malignancy.

a) Mammogram, cranio-
caudad view.

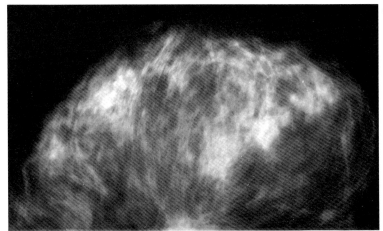

b) Mammogram, mediolateral
view.

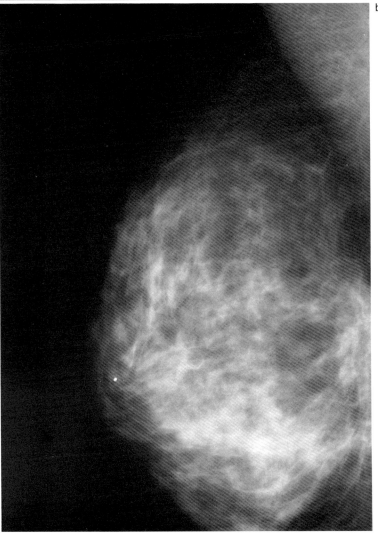

Fig. 38

c) Representative precontrast image of the mammographically suspicious area (arrows) (FLASH 3D: TR = 40 ms, TE = 14 ms, FA = 50°).

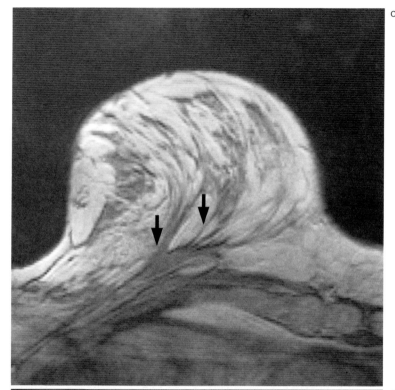

c

d) Postcontrast image (same slice, same pulse sequence) exhibits no significant enhancement, compatible with scarring. No sign of malignancy.

Diagnosis was confirmed by follow-up.

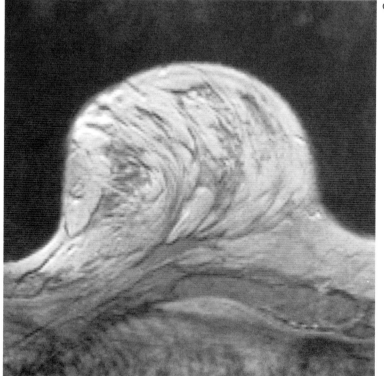

d

Fig. 39

Scarring

Figs. 39a–f
Carcinoma within a breast with extensive scarring after complicated healing. Patient with palpable thickening and mammographically suspicious starlike mass and retraction in the area of previous extensive scarring (first mammogram 5 years after surgery). Since the patient insisted that no change had occurred since surgery and complicated healing, MRI was performed.

a) Mammogram, craniocaudad view.
b) Mammogram, mediolateral view.

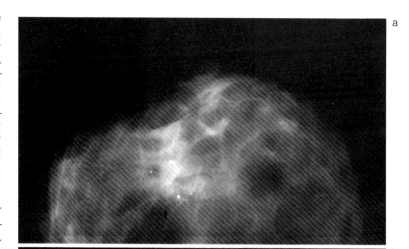

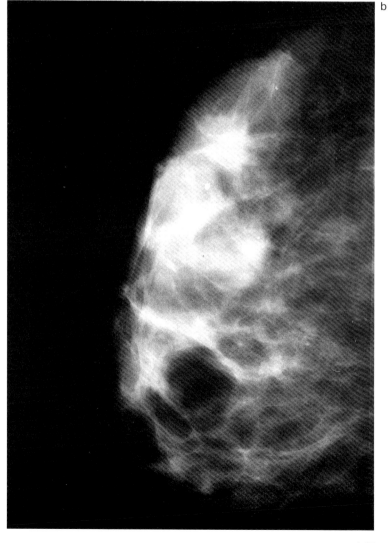

Fig. 39

c) Precontrast scan at the level of the scar (representative slice of a FLASH 3D study: TR = 40 ms, TE = 14 ms, FA = 50°).

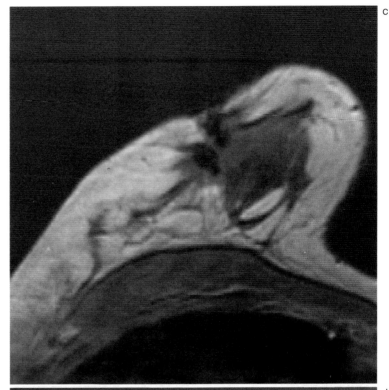

c

d) Postcontrast image demonstrates significant enhancement within this area (arrows), (same slice, same pulse sequence). Signal voids (SV), as shown here, have frequently been encountered within scarring and may be caused by microscopic remnants of metallic glove powder.

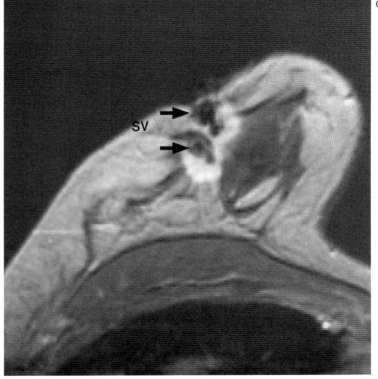

d

Fig. 39   Scarring

e) Further precontrast scan of the same study at another level.

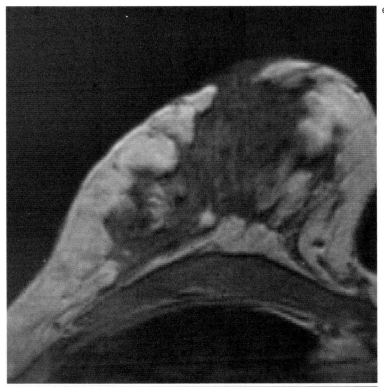

f) Postcontrast image at the same level as e) shows another suspicious enhancing lesion (arrow).

Thus MRI confirmed the suspected carcinoma and indicated multifocal growth.

Histology proved this diagnosis: multifocal ductal carcinoma.

from (51)

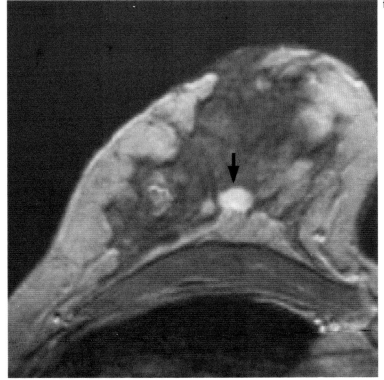

Fig. 40

Figs. 40a–c
Oil cyst in a patient examined for other reasons. The oil cyst (arrows) – already mammographically observed – displays high signal intensity before the administration of Gd-DTPA, which is compatible with its oily contents. After Gd-DTPA neither its wall nor its contents enhance.

a) Mammogram.

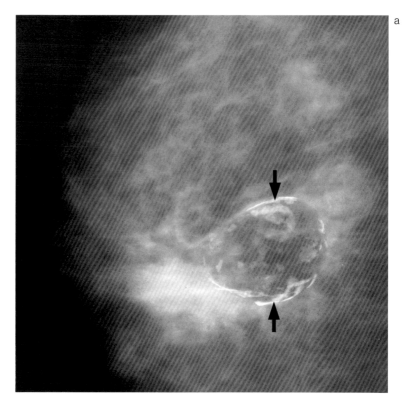

a

Fig. 40   Scarring

b) Precontrast MR image of the oil cyst (SE: TR = 500 ms, TE = 23 ms).

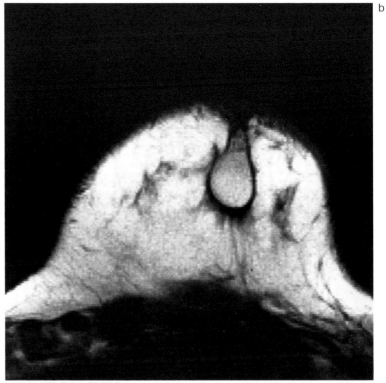

c) Postcontrast MR image (same slice, same pulse sequence).

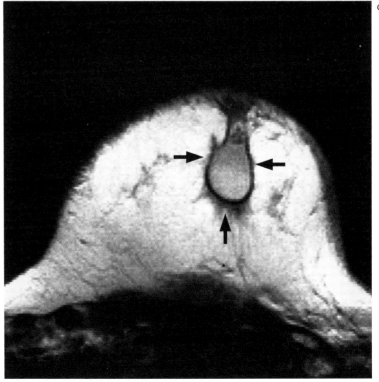

Fig. 41

Figs. 41a–d
Small area of fat necrosis
mimicking malignancy.
In this patient, 18 months
after excision of a mammographically suspicious area,
which histologically had
proven to be proliferative
dysplasia, a new irregular
masslike lesion (arrow) was
detected by mammography
within the scar.

a) Mammogram, cranio-
caudad view.

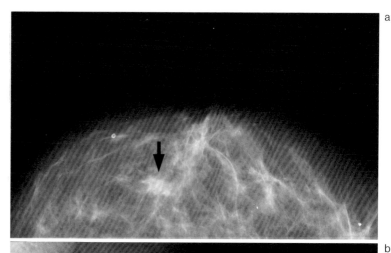

b) Mammogram, mediolateral
view.

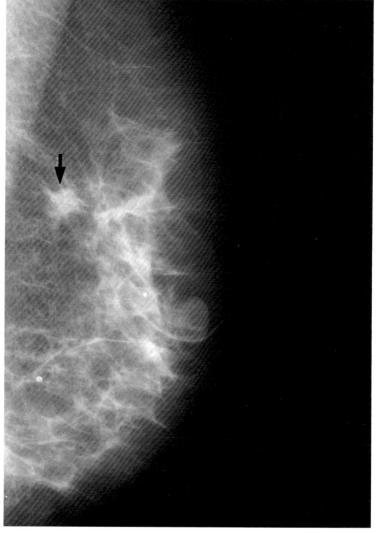

Fig. 41   Scarring

c) Precontrast MR image of the lesion (one of 32 slices of FLASH 3D: TR = 40 ms, TE = 14 ms, FA = 50°).

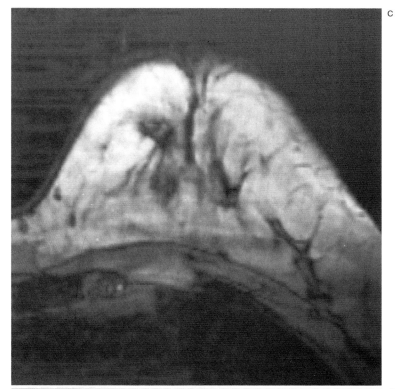

c

d) Postcontrast MR image (same slice, same pulse sequence) shows significant enhancement of the suspicious lesion (arrows). Therefore biopsy was recommended.

Histology: fresh fat necrosis.

In retrospect, the relatively high signal intensity within the lesion on the precontrast scan (comparable to that of surrounding fat) could have been a hint as to its etiology (oily contents). Reliability of such an observation, however, is still uncertain (compare Fig. 42).

from (50)

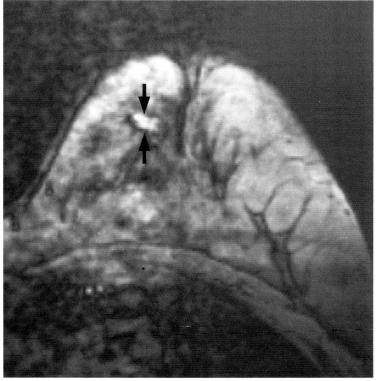

d

Fig. 42

Figs. 42a–c
Carcinoma (diameter 5 mm) behind a silicon implant. The patient presented for MRI with a questionable discrete palpable thickening behind the implant. Neither three-view mammography nor sonography, both performed before MRI, had shown a lesion.

a) Mammogram, cranio-caudad view.

b) On the T1-weighted MR image, however, a small irregular lesion (arrows) was clearly visualized in the area of the palpable abnormality. Contrast agent, which could have further improved specificity, was not yet available at the time of this study.

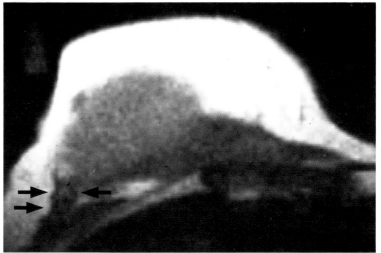

c) Sonographically, it was only possible to demonstrate the small lesion adjacent to the implant (arrows) after meticulous search in retrospect.

Histology: Small ductal carcinoma. The small area of higher signal intensity within the carcinoma (b) histologically corresponded to a tiny island of included fat within the tumor.

from (44a)

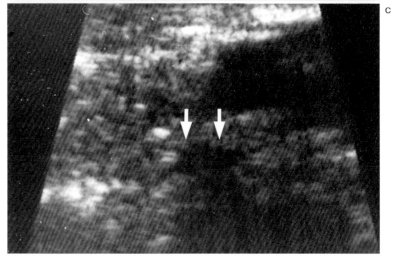

Fig. 43   Scarring with silicon implants

Figs. 43a, b
Recurrence behind an im-
plant with chest wall invasion.
The lesion was already clinically obvious.

a) Precontrast MR image
(representative scan of
FLASH 3D study: TR = 40 ms,
TE = 14 ms, FA = 50°).

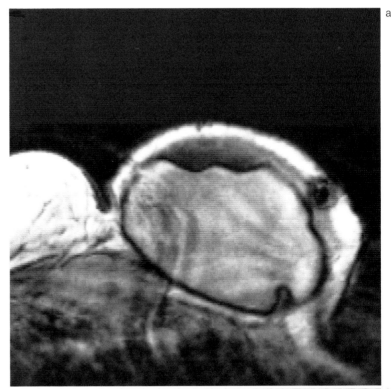

b) Postcontrast image (same
slice, same pulse sequence)
showing significant en-
hancement within the extensive recurrence (arrows).

from (50)

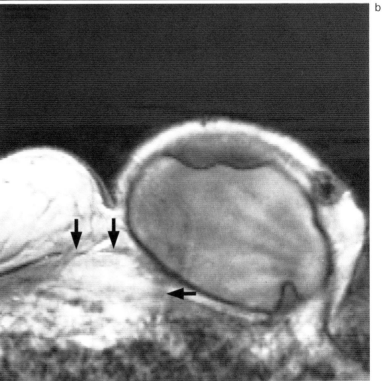

Fig. 44

Figs. 44a–e
Recurrent lobular carcinoma in situ (LCIS) beside the implant visible on MRI alone. MRI was offered to this asymptomatic patient one year after subcutaneous mastectomy and silicon implant because of LCIS as an additional method to evaluate the breast tissue around the implant.

a) Mammogram, craniocaudad view.

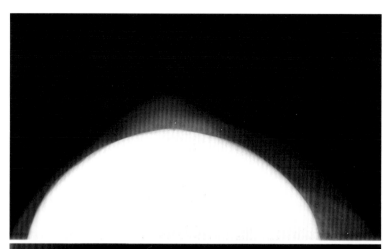

b) Mammogram, mediolateral view. Mammography shows some remaining breast tissue behind the nipple and the scarring. No sign of malignancy, no microcalcifications.

Fig. 44

Scarring with silicon implants

c) Precontrast transverse MR image (FLASH 3D: TR = 40 ms, TE = 14 ms, FA = 50°) shows the implant and the nipple with some remaining retroareolar breast tissue. (F = retroareolar fat)

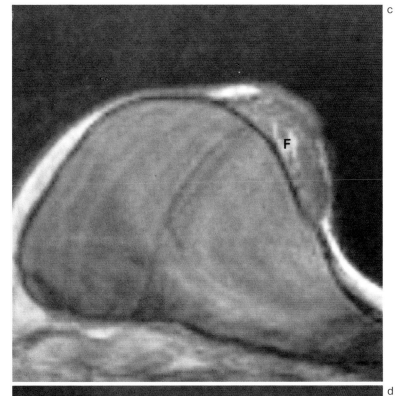

c

d) Corresponding postcontrast image (same slice, same pulse sequence), obtained directly after injection of Gd-DTPA (minute 0–5). Whereas retroareolar fat (F) and breast tissue do not enhance significantly, a suspicious slowly enhancing area was noted lateral to the implant (arrows).

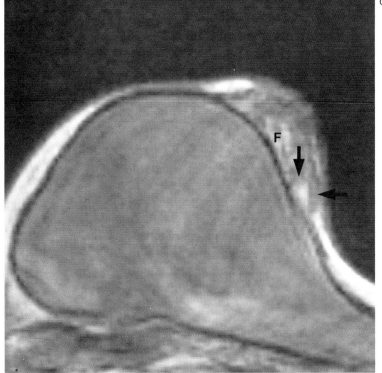

d

Fig. 44

e) Second postcontrast image, obtained in a second 3D measurement (minute 7–12). Since phase- and frequency-encoding gradients were not exchanged for this measurement, motion artifacts of the heart cross the medial parts of the breast. Whereas retroareolar fat (F) and breast tissue do not enhance significantly, the suspicious slowly enhancing area is seen lateral to the implant (arrows). It was removed after MR-guided needle localization and proved to be a small area of recurrent LCIS.

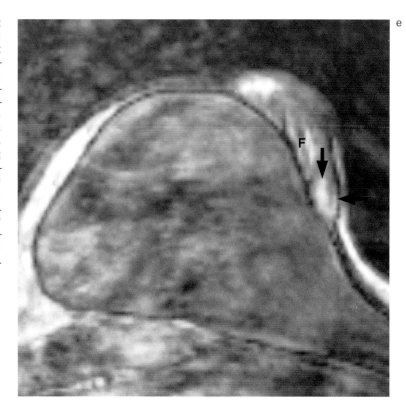

e

Fig. 45

Scarring with silicon implants

Figs. 45a–d
Large granuloma beside an implant.
Ten years after reconstructive surgery because of breast cancer, the patient presented with a large palpable mass, which she had first noticed about 6 months before. Malignancy could not be excluded mammographically or sonographically.

a) Craniocaudad mammogram showing the dense mass beside the implant.

a

b) Sonogram demonstrating a shadowing lesion, which is barely penetrated.

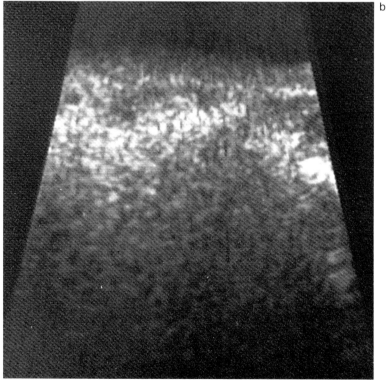

b

Fig. 45

c) Precontrast MR image of the lesion (arrows) beside the implant (arrowheads) (SE: TR = 500 ms, TE = 30 ms).

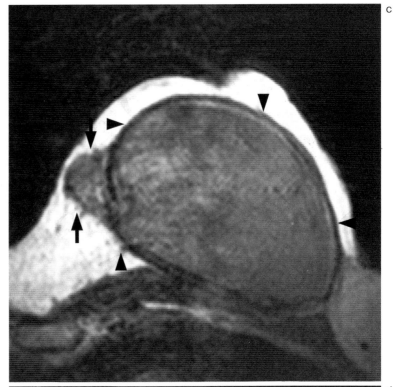

d) Postcontrast image (same slice, same pulse sequence) shows very little nonsignificant enhancement within the lesion, strongly suggesting benign etiology.

Because of the limited experience with MRI at the time of this study, biopsy was nevertheless performed.

Histology: granuloma with silicon inclusions.

from (46)

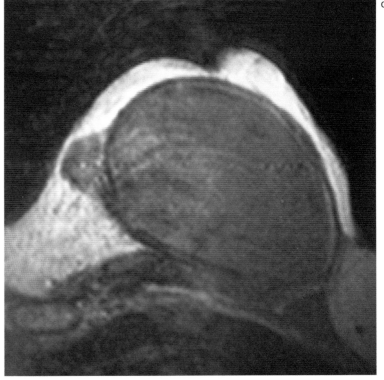

Status after limited surgery and radiation therapy (RT)

Conservative treatment of breast cancer has become an important new method. Diagnostic evaluation of scarring within the irradiated breast is, however, usually even more difficult than within the nonirradiated breast. Besides a frequently more pronounced local scarring, increased generalized fibrosis (caused by the radiation) and sometimes fat necrosis may obscure or mimic malignancy (13, 44, 61, 98, 103, 114).

Clinically – after regression of initial swelling within about the first 18 months – thickening of skin and breast tissue frequently persists in varying degrees. This fact makes evaluation more difficult.

Mammographic evaluation within about the first 18 months after radiation is frequently impaired by increased overall density, decreased compressibility from swelling, and pronounced changes around the scar. Later on – besides the frequently pronounced changes around the scar itself – postradiation fibrosis may be responsible for thickening of ligaments, persisting overall density and sometimes retraction. Typical ringlike calcifications and also indeterminate microcalcifications may occur within smaller areas of fat necrosis. Larger areas of fat necrosis may cause masses which, because of their irregular contours, are clinically and mammographically indistinguishable from malignancy.

Sonography performed at regular intervals has proven helpful in evaluating these posttreatment breasts. Because of fibrosis, the echogenicity of the irradiated tissue usually increases, allowing good contrast with most malignancies, which display lower echogenicity. Nevertheless, unless regular follow-up studies exist, the differential diagnosis of shadowing and hypoechoic areas, which might be caused by either scarring or malignancy, proves quite difficult. In addition, the limited capabilities of ultrasound in excluding early malignancy must again be considered.

On MRI (41), shortly after RT (month 0–6) significant enhancement with a fast rise of signal intensity after the injection of Gd-DTPA is usually encountered in the irradiated tissue. This enhancement may be diffuse throughout the complete breast tissue or it may be more pronounced in areas with relatively higher radiation dosage (in the parasternal region if a sternal field was used, or in both medial and lateral parts of large breasts, for example) or around the scar. Such large areas with diffuse enhancement are probably composed of numerous tiny areas of increased microvascular fragility after treatment, which contain multiple small fat necroses (Fig. 46 a, b). Focal, large, strongly enhancing areas of fat necrosis have occurred in 2 of 60 patients we examined after RT (Fig. 47). Because of their strong enhancement, neither early changes after RT nor fresh fat necrosis can be distinguished from malignancy.

Starting about 6 months after RT (month 7–18), both amount and speed of enhancement decrease slowly with time, but with remarkable individual variations. Therefore, toward the end of this period (month 12-18), distinction between malignancy and postradiation changes improves, depending on the individual amount of posttreatment changes. Therefore, during this time malignancy can be excluded in cases where little or no enhancement is present. Diffuse or focal enhancement, however, can be caused by both malignancy and posttreatment changes. Therefore, whenever positive enhancement (focal or diffuse) exists within an otherwise suspicious area, biopsy remains necessary for further diagnosis (Fig. 48). Dynamic imaging or any other method of imaging very early after Gd-DTPA may help to distinguish the early enhancing types of carcinomas from radiation changes with a more delayed enhancement. However, this distinction is not completely reliable.

18 months and later after RT no significant enhancement usually exists within the irradiated tissue, which indicates completion of the inflammatory, reactive, and fibrotic reaction. Due to the very slight enhancement seen within the irradiated tissue, both exclusion and detection of malignancy then are excellent (Figs. 49 through 52) and contrast-enhanced MRI offers significant additional information compared to the other methods.

Figure 52 summarizes the change of enhancement with time compared to the enhancement seen in malignancy and recurrences. Individual variations observed in our patients are indicated by the standard deviation.

In summary, contrast-enhanced MRI can provide significant additional information within mammographically dense and distorted tissue later than 18 months after radiation therapy (41, 79). Provided a lesion smaller than the slice thickness is excluded (small group of microcalcifications), we meanwhile rely on the MRI examination if no or little enhancement exists (even in the presence of questionable palpable abnormalities, mammographic distortion, or masslike fibrosis). Focal enhancement may allow earlier detection of malignancy than the other methods, even though focal fat necrosis or other tumors have to be considered as well. Diffuse enhancement, which does not exclude malignancy, was rare later than 18 months after therapy in our group of patients, all treated with 50 Gy megavoltage X-ray and cobalt therapy and with 10 Gy electron boost*.

Between 12 and 18 months after therapy, contrast-enhanced MRI might be tried in diagnostically difficult cases. Here again, no enhancement excludes malignancy; positive enhancement needs close correlation with other methods.

Earlier than 12 months after RT, MRI is usually not helpful due to the strong underlying enhancement. It is therefore not recommended during that time span.

* Different enhancement behavior might be encountered after interstitial radiation therapy.

Fig. 46

Figs. 46a–d
Change of enhancement
behavior with time after radiation therapy (RT).
On the first MRI study, performed 9 months after RT (a, b),
significant diffuse en-
hancement is encountered
within the complete breast
tissue. On the second MRI
study of the same breast,
performed 18 months after RT
(c, d), no significant enhancement is visible any more.

a) First study: precontrast
image (FLASH 3D:
TR = 40 ms, TE = 14 ms,
FA = 50°).

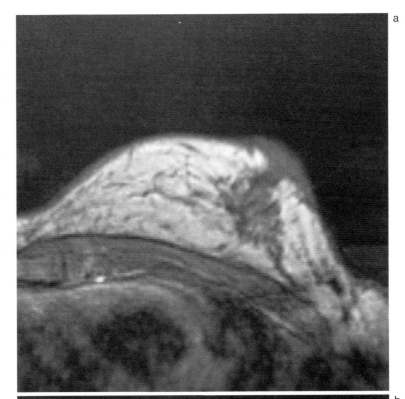

a

b) First study: postcontrast
image (same slice, same
pulse sequence).

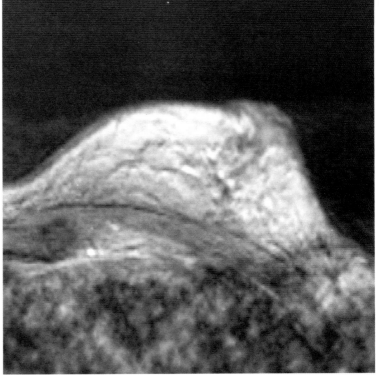

b

Fig. 46

Status after RT

c) Second study: precontrast image (similar slice as a), same pulse sequence).

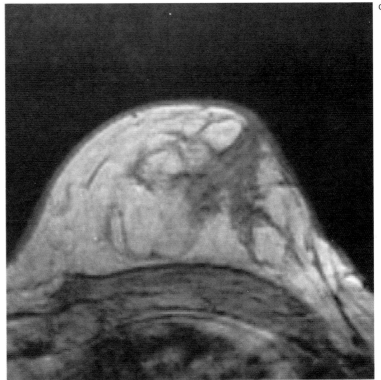

d) Second study: postcontrast image (same slice as c), same pulse sequence).

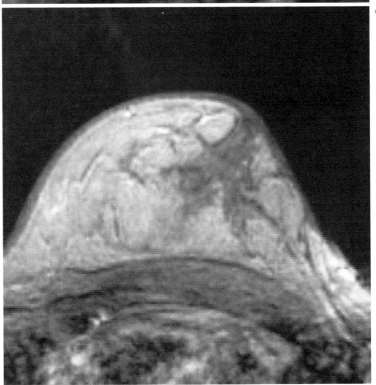

Fig. 47

Figs. 47a, b
Fat necrosis within the scar in the parasternal region 8 months post RT. RT had included the usual tangential breast fields and a sternal field.

a) Precontrast scan at the clinically and mammographically suspicious area (FLASH 2D: TR = 30 ms, TE = 13 ms, FA = 50°).

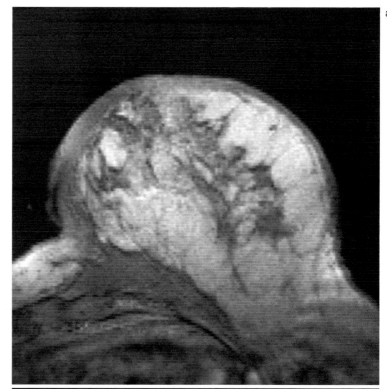
a

b) Postcontrast scan, obtained 3 minutes post i.v. injection of Gd-DTPA (same slice, same pulse sequence), shows irregular tissue medially which enhances significantly (arrow). Furthermore, pronounced partially enhancing skin thickening is noticed in the medial breast (arrowheads).

Histology: fat necrosis.

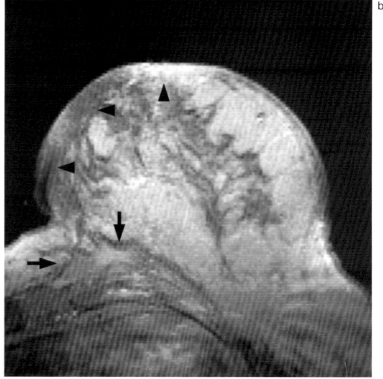
b

Fig. 48   Status after RT

Figs. 48a–d
Recurrent carcinoma within a
diffusely enhancing breast
15 months post RT.
The patient presented with a
swollen breast and a pal-
pable mass beside the nipple
15 months post RT.

a) Mammogram cranio-
caudad view.

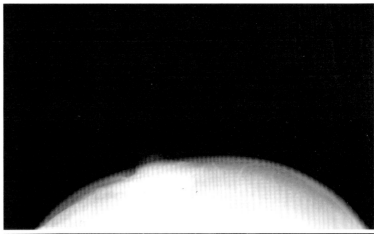

b) Mammogram, mediolateral
view.

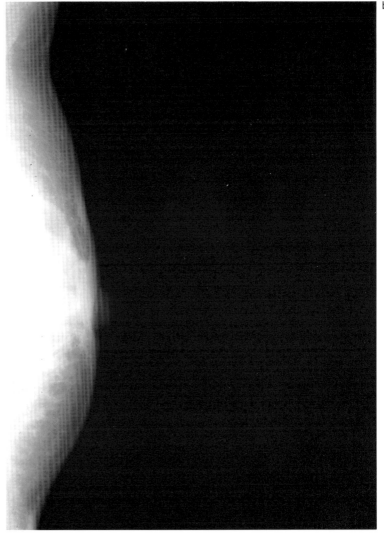

Fig. 48

c) Precontrast MR image at the level of the palpable mass (arrow) (FLASH 3D: TR = 40 ms, TE = 14 ms, FA = 50°).

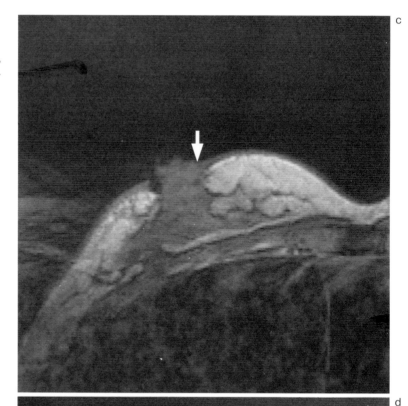

d) Postcontrast MR image (same slice, same pulse sequence) shows significant enhancement both within the palpable mass (arrows) and the surrounding tissue.

Even though these findings were initially interpreted as unsuspicious by an unexperienced examiner, biopsy was performed. Biopsy confirmed the mass to be recurrent tumor. No further tumor was found within the surrounding enhancing tissue.

This case emphasizes that in the presence of diffuse enhancement carcinoma can never be excluded. Therefore, further investigation of any otherwise suspicious area (palpable mass or mammographically suspicious lesion) is necessary.

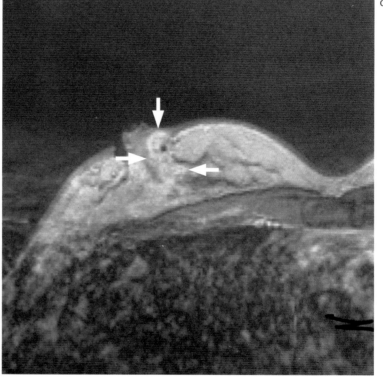

Fig. 49   Status after RT

Figs. 49a–d
Multifocal recurrence
15 months after RT.
The patient presented with
nipple discharge and a swollen breast. A routine mammogram, which showed a
group of microcalcifications
(arrow) in the retroareolar
area, had been obtained
2 months previously and the
changes at that time were
interpreted as postradiation
changes.

a) Mammogram, craniocaudad view.

b) Mammogram, mediolateral
view.

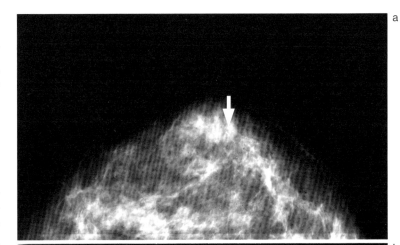

a

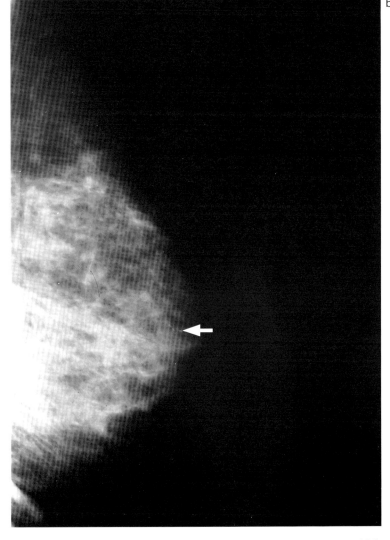

b

Fig. 49

c) Representative precontrast image at the level of the nipple (one of 32 images of a FLASH 3D study: TR = 40 ms, TE = 14 ms, FA = 50°).

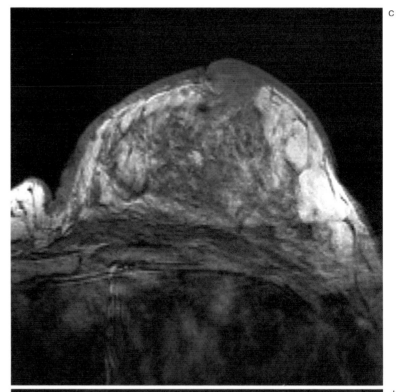

c

d) Postcontrast MR image (same slice, same pulse sequence) shows strong ringlike enhancement around the nipple as well as another ringlike enhancing focus centrally. Several more foci were detected on further slices, suggesting multifocal recurrence.

Histology: multifocal recurrence of undifferentiated carcinoma with central necrosis within the foci.

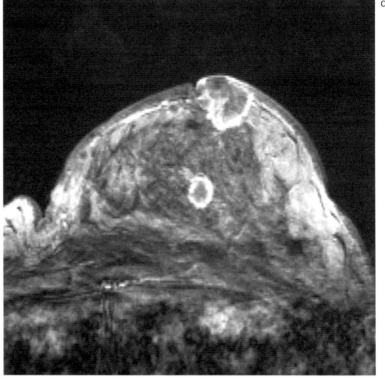

d

Fig. 50

Status after RT

Figs. 50a–d
Extensive posttreatment changes, posing diagnostic problems.
This patient presented with a large suspicious area of thickening at about 3 o'clock laterally in the left breast, 30 months after excision and RT of a breast carcinoma and 12 months after excision of recurrent tumor and chemotherapy. Mammographically malignancy could not be excluded within the dense tissue.

a) Mammogram, craniocaudad view.

b) Mammogram, mediolateral view.

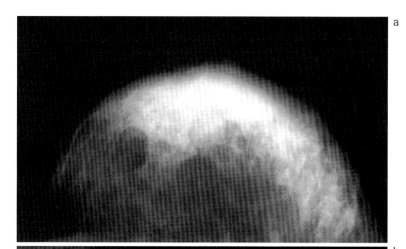

a

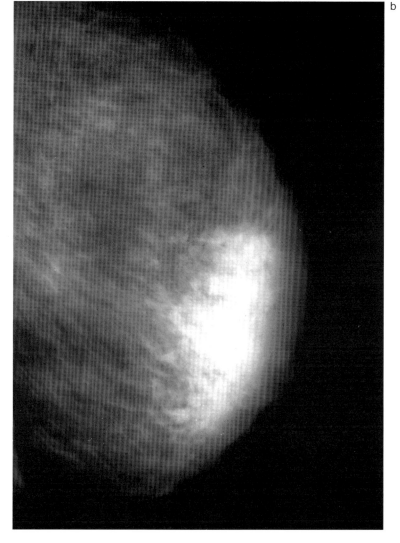

b

Fig. 50

c) Precontrast image (one representative of 32 slices of a FLASH 3D study: TR = 40 ms, TE = 14 ms, FA = 50°).

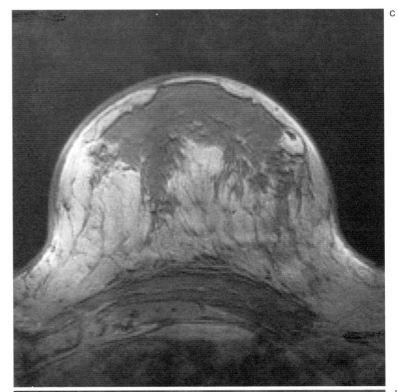

c

d) Postcontrast image (same slice, same pulse sequence) demonstrates irregular and dense fibrotic tissue and moderate skin thickening. Based on absent enhancement, malignancy was excluded.

Biopsy was nevertheless later on performed because of the strong clinical suspicion and confirmed post treatment fibrosis.

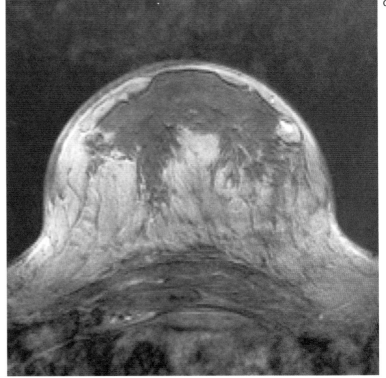

d

Fig. 51   Status after RT

Figs. 51a–f
Recurrence detected by MRI alone.
This patient was examined by MRI 26 months after RT in a study in which all patients with dense tissue after tumorectomy and RT were offered an MRI examination. No palpable abnormality and no expressible nipple discharge were detected, even in retrospect knowing the result of the MRI examination. Mammography shows a starlike density central within the breast (arrowhead), which had regressed since the previous examination 1 year before and thus represents scarring.

a) Craniocaudad mammogram, 1 year before the examination.

b) Craniocaudad mammogram at the time of the examination.

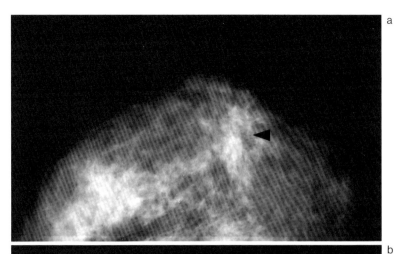

a

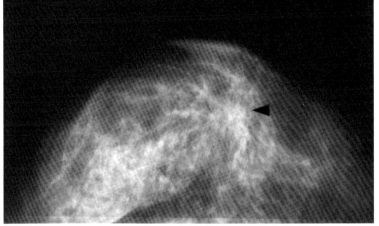

b

Fig. 51

c) Precontrast MR image at the level of the scar (FLASH 3D: TR = 40 ms, TE = 14 ms, FA = 50°).

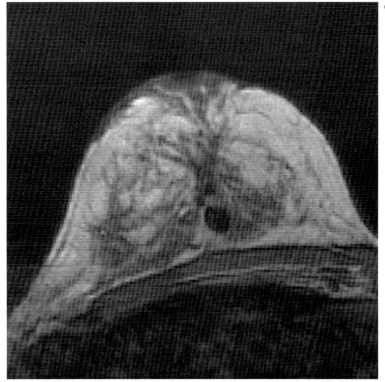

c

d) The postcontrast MR image (same slice, same pulse sequence) demonstrates the starlike scar (arrowhead), which does not enhance. Behind the scar close to the chest wall and adjacent to a nonenhancing cyst (cy), however, a strongly enhancing highly suspicious lesion (arrow) is visualized.

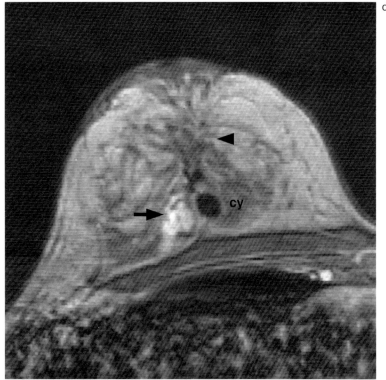

d

Fig. 51   Status after RT

e) Neighboring precontrast slice through the nipple (same pulse sequence).

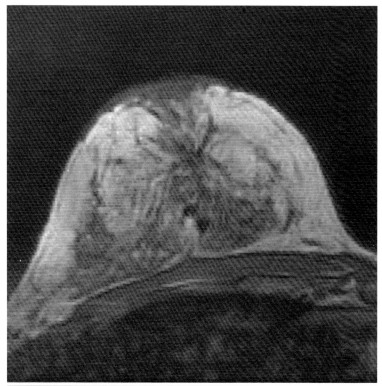

f) Postcontrast image of this neighboring slice shows another independent suspicious enhancement within the retromammillar ducts (arrow).

MR-guided biopsy of the two lesions suspicious on MRI confirmed a 1.1 cm mucinous invasive recurrent tumor close to the chest wall (c, d) and a second intraductal carcinoma independent of the first within the retromammillar ducts (e, f).

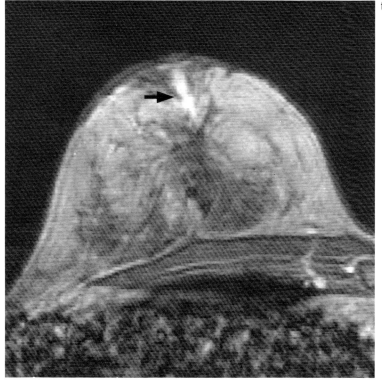

Fig. 52

Fig. 52
Amount of enhancement after irradiation.
The amount of enhancement (mean ± single standard deviation) was measured in the irradiated tissue in 60 patients after tumorectomy and radiation therapy. (Group A: 0–6 months after RT, Group B: 6–12 months after RT, Group C: 12–18 months after RT, Group D >18 months after RT).

The amount of enhancement relative to the threshold of significance (two different techniques were used: 2D SE and 3D FLASH at 1.0 Tesla) is plotted against time after irradiation. (Thresholds and technique see pages 26–31.)

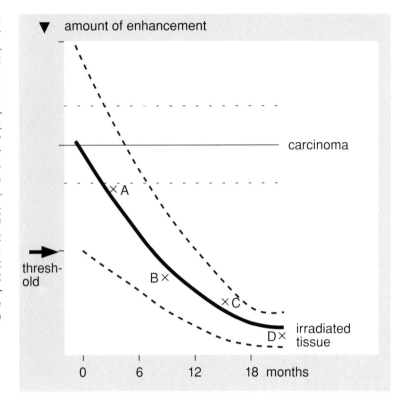

Clinical application of contrast-enhanced MRI

When a method is introduced for clinical application, it is important to assess its accuracy and reliability and to know its advantages and disadvantages. For this reason, current data concerning the accuracy of contrast-enhanced MRI are discussed first (see pages 177–180). On page 182 indications are proposed based on contrast-enhanced MRI's specific advantages and drawbacks. Examples finally demonstrate how we use contrast-enhanced MRI in diagnostically difficult cases.

Accuracy

As already mentioned, present worldwide experience (end of 1989) with contrast-enhanced MRI of the breast includes more than 1,000 examinations. Our experiences, based on more than 500 cases, will be discussed in more detail.

Since contrast-enhanced MRI in all studies has been used and should also further be used as a supplementary noninvasive method, the most accurate and realistic way to assess its value is to compare the diagnoses, which were based on conventional diagnostics (pre-MRI) before MRI was performed, and those based on both conventional diagnostics and MRI (post-MRI) in the same patient.

Considering the known influence of preselection accuracy data are shown for two different groups of our patients (Tables 10 and 11):

The data of all biopsy-proven cases (Table 10) are, of course, the best confirmed. The accuracy of conventional diagnostics in these cases compares well with corresponding data reported in the literature. This group does, however, contain a high number of obvious cases (high prevalence of carcinomas that were true positive pre- and post-MRI anyway), since in 1985 and 1986 MRI was used in as many preoperative cases as possible to gain experience. On the other hand, many patients with negative MRI diagnoses are not considered in this group, because since 1987 the majority of these patients were not biopsied, but followed.

The group of diagnostically difficult patients (Table 11) includes cases examined until the end of 1988 only. These cases are either confirmed by follow-up of at least 12 months

177

a

	pre-MRI	post-MRI
sensitivity	90%	100%
specificity	16%	22%
negative predictive value	58%	100%
positive predictive value	55%	60%

b

histologically proven diagnoses	no. of cases
carcinoma	131
lymphoma	2
"cystosarcoma phylloides"	1
fibroadenoma	35
papilloma	2
nonproliferative dysplasia	11
moderate proliferative dysplasia	40
strong proliferative dysplasia	9
scarring	11
inflammatory	6
others	2

or by biopsy. In this group, the accuracy of conventional diagnostics is not good because of the known preselection, including only those cases where conventional diagnosis was impaired (mammographically dense breast, extensive scarring, etc.). Nevertheless, this group best represents the majority of patients presently examined by MRI at our institution. It also best represents the group of patients for whom MRI is recommended (see indications, page 181).

As shown by Tables 10 and 11, sensitivity and negative predictive value of MRI are excellent for both groups of patients. This finding corresponds to MRI's ability to detect otherwise unknown lesions (especially within dense breast tissue) and to its high value for exclusion of malignancy in cases of non-significant enhancement.

Specificity and positive predictive value in the group of biopsy-proven cases (Table 10) are only slightly higher for

Table 11a, b	pre-MRI	post-MRI	a
sensitivity	74%	100%	
specificity	32%	53%	
negative predictive value	85%	100%	
positive predictive value	19%	31%	

Accuracy in diagnostically difficult cases.

a) Accuracy in 192 diagnostically difficult cases: The pre-MRI diagnoses, based on mammography, clinical examination and sonography (if necessary) are compared with the post-MRI diagnoses, based on the above-mentioned methods and MRI. All diagnoses were established preoperatively.

b) The histologic findings of the above-shown 192 diagnoses are listed.

diagnosis	no. of cases	biopsy-proven cases		b
carcinoma	34	34		
fibroadenoma	16	10		
papilloma	4	1		
nonenhancing dysplasia	55	8	nonproliferative dysplasia	
enhancing dysplasia	48	24	moderate proliferative dysplasia	
		8	strong proliferative dysplasia	
scarring	25	7		
inflammatory	9	6		
others	1	0		

post-MRI than for pre-MRI diagnoses. This fact and the relatively low specificity of both pre- and post-MRI diagnostics in this group are influenced by the low prevalence of nonenhancing lesions (25 out of 250) compared to the high number of enhancing lesions (225 out of 250), for which biopsy had to be recommended since no certain criteria for further distinction exist with any method (e.g., differential diagnosis: carcinoma versus fibroadenoma).

In diagnostically difficult cases (Table 11), for comparison, specificity and positive predictive value are superior for the post-MRI diagnoses than the pre-MRI diagnoses. This finding is explained by the noticeably higher number of nonenhancing lesions (83 out of 192), for which MRI was able to exclude malignancy in this population.

Summarizing the results of accuracy data in the different groups, the value of MRI in case of absent enhancement is further confirmed. In case of focal enhancement further investigation (including biopsy) is indicated, since MRI's high sensitivity offers the chance of detecting additional lesions. The specificity of this finding is comparable to (Table 10 and 11) the corresponding specificity of conventional diagnostics. In case of diffuse enhancement MRI does not offer advantages over conventional imaging.

Thus these statistical data confirm the proposed guidelines for further work-up based on MRI findings (pages 50, 51).

When accuracy data of the literature (16, 66, 70, 79, 82, 113, 117) are analyzed, they agree very well with our data:

The three false negative calls so far reported in the literature can all be explained by methodology. Two carcinomas were not included in the imaging volume in a dynamic study of selected slices only (66) or in an examination with 2D SE technique and gaps between the slices (82). One more carcinoma of 5 mm was significantly smaller than the slice thickness of 10 mm used (82). We have experienced similar problems, especially with SE technique in one borderline case (see Fig. 29).

The described false negative calls emphasize the importance of optimum technique. Furthermore, MRI interpretation should be confined to lesions larger than the slice thickness used, which is usually counterchecked by mammography.

The percentage of false positive calls reported by the other authors is even lower than ours. This was achieved by using delayed speed of enhancement or well-circumscribed enhancement as criteria of benignity. Both increase specificity from fewer false positive calls (concerning, e.g., fibroadenomas or proliferative dysplasias). However, since rare carcinomas with delayed or well-circumscribed enhancement might thus be misdiagnosed, we do not recommend using these criteria (see also page 49). Such a policy may increase specificity at the cost of the excellent sensitivity, which to us appears a unique advantage of this method.

In summary, excellent data concerning the accuracy of contrast-enhanced MRI already exist. By and large these data agree very well and strongly support the value of MRI. Nevertheless, further investigations to increase the present data base are desirable.

Indications

Since MRI is still a quite expensive and relatively complicated method (requiring special equipment like the breast coil, interpretation of almost 100 tomographic images per breast, and examination time of about 30 minutes), it should be used in selected cases only.

Indications for its use result from the weak points of conventional breast diagnostics (see pages 12–15) and from the advantages of contrast-enhanced MRI.

Advantages of MRI include the tomographic technique, which allows assessment of tissues without superimposition (especially important in dense breast tissue and behind silicon implants), complete visualization of the breast tissue even close to the chest wall, and finally the excellent distinction between nonenhancing tissues (such as scarring, nonenhancing dysplasias, normal breast tissue, and cysts) and enhancing lesions (such as malignant but also benign tumors). Due to its excellent negative predictive value and sensitivity, MRI is uniquely valuable for the exclusion of malignancy. Finally, it offers the chance of detecting a previously unknown lesion, above all within dense tissue, because of its very high sensitivity. Compared to computerized tomography the significantly higher sensitivity of MRI for contrast medium, the excellent tolerance of Gd-DTPA (95a), and the absence of the significant radiation dose applied to the breast by CT are major advantages.

Disadvantages center around the limited information of diffuse enhancement. Therefore, MRI is not recommended if proliferative dysplasia, microcalcifications, secretory disease, or inflammatory changes are known to exist.

Because MRI is a tomographic technique, partial volume effect may also influence the evaluation. Therefore, MRI interpretation should be limited to lesions larger than or in the range of the slice thickness. This caveat usually creates no problems, because MRI should be applied as an additional tool in any case. Close correlation with the other modalities also minimizes the theoretical risk of overlooking an enhancement or mistaking enhancement for a vessel or vice versa, when about 100 images per breast have to be interpreted.

Based on the discussed advantages and limitations, contrast-enhanced MRI should be used with other modalities. Under these circumstances, it has proven to offer valuable additional information for the following indications:

– Differentiation of irregularly shaped densities.

– Differentiation of asymmetric tissues.

– Exclusion of malignancy within mammographically very dense tissue (e.g., questionable palpable findings, search for primary tumor, exclusion of further malignancy when limited surgery of a small malignancy is planned).

– Distinction between extensive scarring and malignancy ($>$6 months postoperative or $>$18 months after RT).

– Supplementary evaluation of patients with silicon implants.

Figures 53 through 71 demonstrate how we apply MRI in diagnostically difficult cases. Its application in cases with scarring, silicon implants, or after radiation therapy has already been treated extensively on pages 138–176. The major guidelines for interpretation are outlined on pages 50 and 51.

As shown by these examples, when applied in selected diagnostically difficult cases, MRI cannot, of course, solve all problems, but in many cases it offers valuable and frequently decisive additional information (49).

Fig. 53   Indications

Figs. 53a–e
Mammographically dense breast and questionable palpable abnormality. The patient presented with an uncertain palpable thickening in the upper outer quadrant and mammographically quite dense tissue. Even though sonography showed a suspicious small hypoechoic area in this region, further confirmation was desired because of the uncertain palpable findings.

a) Craniocaudad mammogram.
b) Mediolateral mammogram.

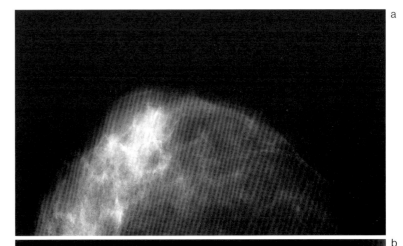

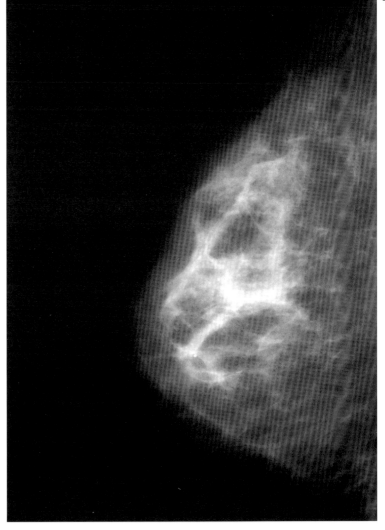

Fig. 53

c) Precontrast MR image (one of 32 slices of a FLASH 3D study: TR = 40 ms, TE = 14 ms, FA = 50°).

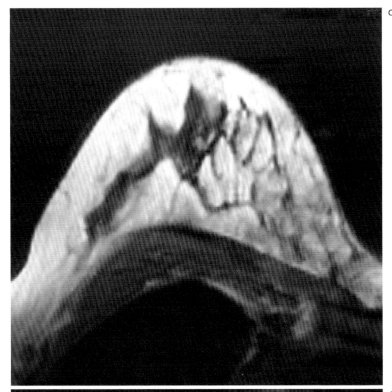

c

d) Postcontrast MR image (same slice, same pulse sequence) confirms an irregular strongly enhancing lesion in the clinically and sonographically suspicious area (arrow).

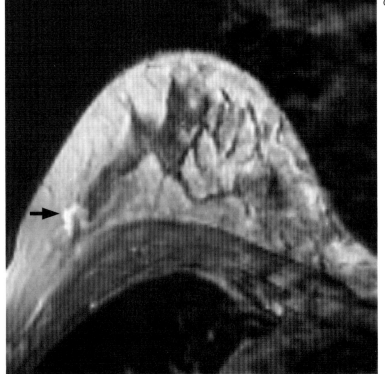

d

Fig. 53   Indications

e) Sonography.

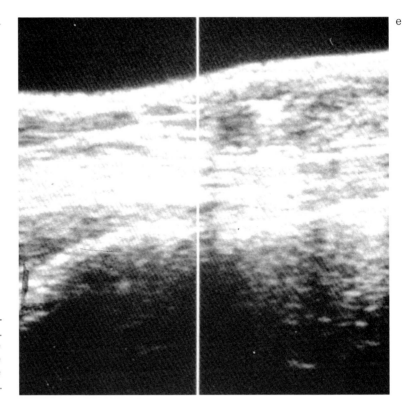

e

Histology: 1 cm predomi-
nantly mucinous carcinoma.
The mucinous nature of the
carcinoma may explain the
uncharacteristic palpable
findings.

Fig. 54

Figs. 54a–d
This patient presented with a very lumpy breast and a sonographically questionable hypoechoic area at 6 o'clock.

a) With the dense breast tissue, containing multiple diffuse microcalcifications, malignancy could not be positively excluded.

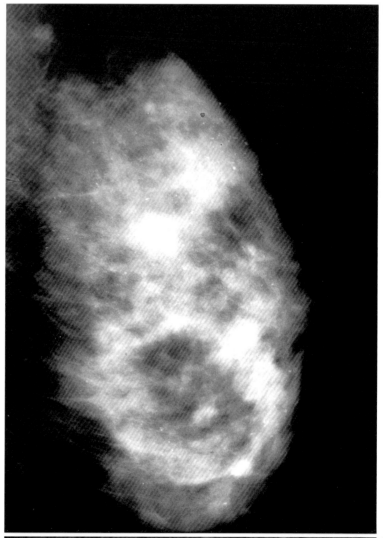

a

b) Sonographically, even with selective compression a reliable distinction between fat lobule and malignancy appeared impossible.

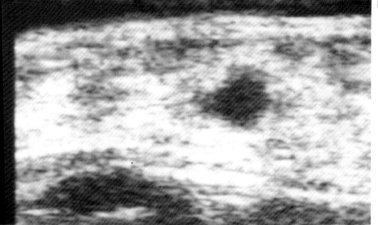

b

Fig. 54
Indications

c) Precontrast transverse MR image at the level of the sonographic findings (FLASH 3D: TR = 40 ms, TE = 14 ms, FA = 50°).

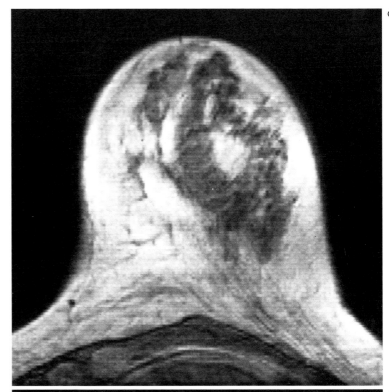

c

d) Postcontrast MR image (same slice, same pulse sequence) exhibits no enhancement.

Based on absent enhancement within the complete breast tissue, malignancy was excluded and follow-up recommended by MRI.

Diagnosis: dysplastic tissue, confirmed by follow-up and finally by biopsy 1 year later.

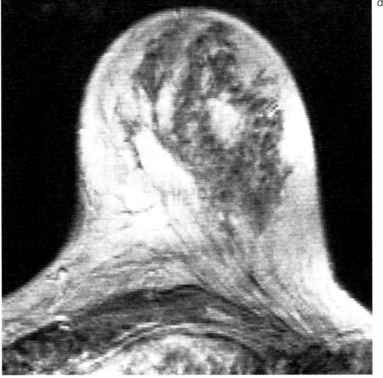

d

Fig. 55

Figs. 55a–e
Mammographically dense breast and questionable palpable abnormality. The patient presented with a questionable slight thickening in the upper outer quadrant within mammographically dense tissue. Due to multiple small hypoechoic areas, sonography was equivocal. MRI was requested to exclude malignancy, since the palpable findings were considered subtle.

a) Mammogram, craniocaudad view.

b) Mammogram, mediolateral view.

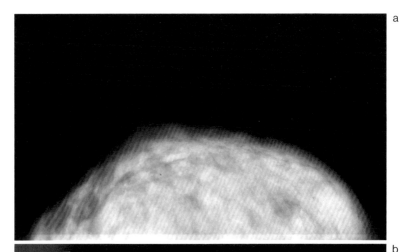

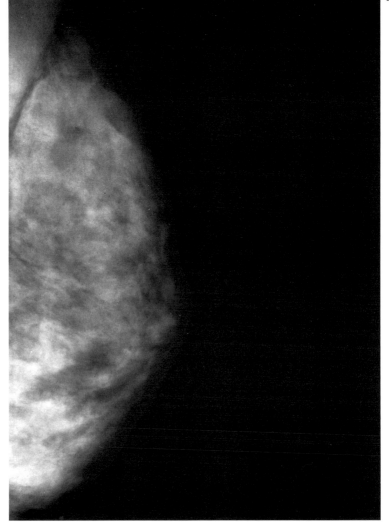

Fig. 55   Indications

c) Precontrast MR image at the area of slight thickening (FLASH 3D: TR = 40 ms, TE = 14 ms, FA = 50°).

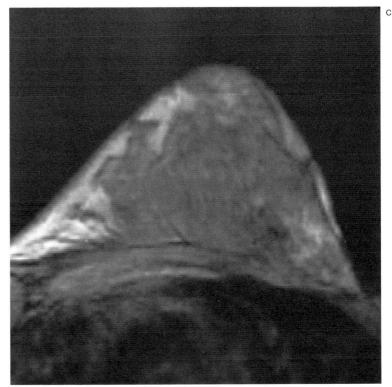

d) Postcontrast MR image (same slice, same pulse sequence) shows strong enhancement in this area (arrows). Therefore, biopsy was strongly recommended.

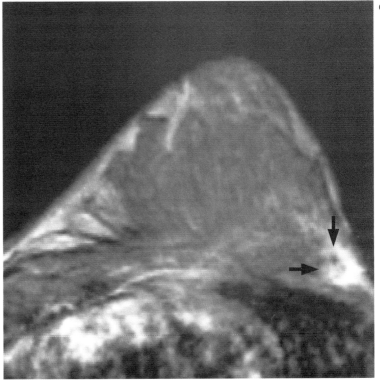

Fig. 55

e) Sonogram.

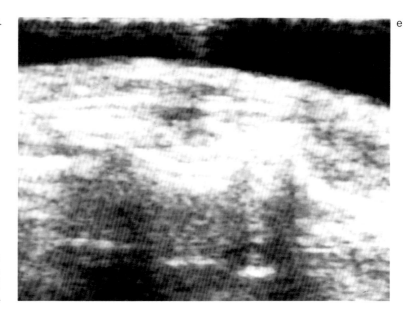

e

Histology: the area proved to consist of local dysplasia with strong proliferation and atypias.

Fig. 56

Indications

Figs. 56a–d
Asymmetry.
The patient presented with moderate palpable and significant mammographic asymmetry, detected on the baseline mammogram. MRI was requested to exclude malignancy.

a) Left mammogram, craniocaudad view, showing prominent asymmetric tissue.

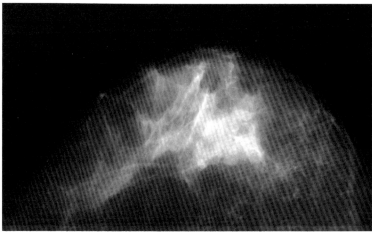

b) Right mammogram, craniocaudad view.

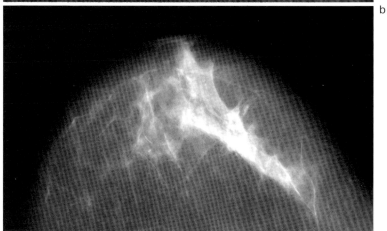

Fig. 56

c) Precontrast MR image (representative slice of 32 images of FLASH 3D: TR = 40 ms, TE = 14 ms, FA = 50°).

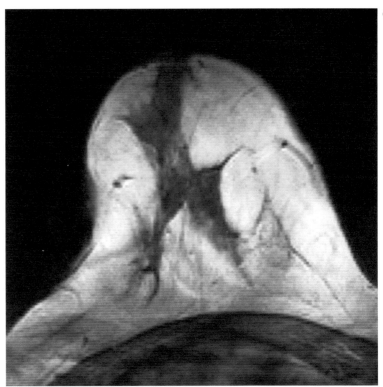

c

d) Postcontrast MR image (same slice, same pulse sequence). The absence of enhancement reliably excludes malignancy within the large asymmetric tissue. Enhancement is visible only within the vessels.

Both the enhancement within the vessels, and the increased intensity of the artifacts (arrowheads) – caused by Gd-DTPA-enhanced blood within the moving heart – are important proofs that Gd-DTPA was injected and arrived. Thus, backward flow of injected Gd-DTPA within the infusion tube into the infusion bottle with NaCl 0.9% caused by an occluded needle can be excluded.

Diagnosis: asymmetric breast tissue, confirmed by 2-year follow-up.

from (72)

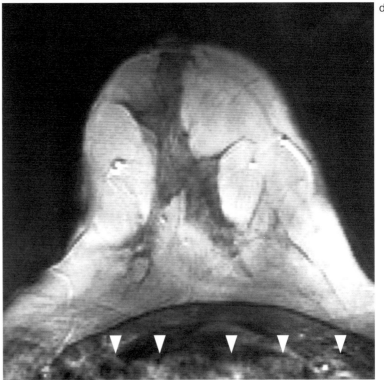

d

Fig. 57

Indications

Figs. 57a–c
Asymmetry.
This patient presented with mammographic and moderate palpable asymmetry known for years, without significant change. Sonography was inconclusive due to multiple small hypoechoic areas.

a) Left and right craniocaudad mammograms.

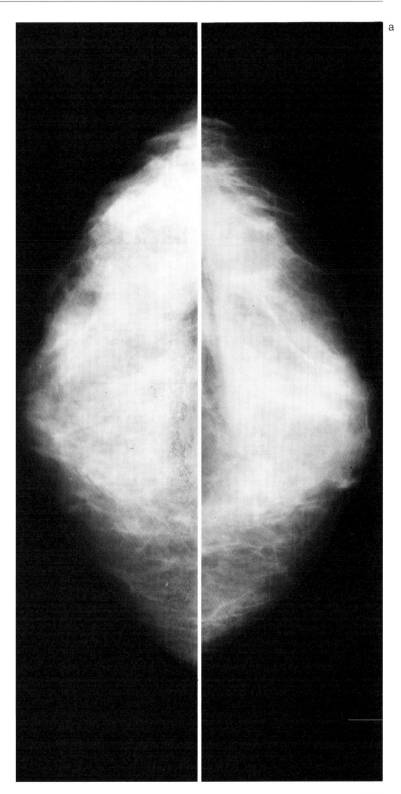

a

Fig. 57

b) Precontrast MR image (representative slice through the outer quadrant; FLASH 2D: TR = 30 ms, TE = 13 ms, FA = 50°).

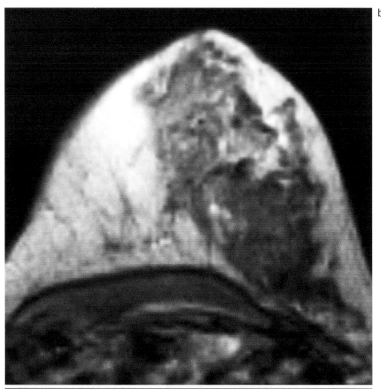

b

c) Postcontrast MR image (same slice, same pulse sequence) shows strong enhancement within the complete upper outer quadrant (arrows). Considering the quite uncharacteristic and unchanged palpable findings, the differential diagnosis predominantly included proliferative dysplasia or diffusely growing barely palpable carcinoma. Therefore, biopsy was strongly recommended.

Histology: extensive lobular carcinoma in situ (corresponding to the MR findings) including a small area of invasive lobular carcinoma (1.5 cm).

from (38a)

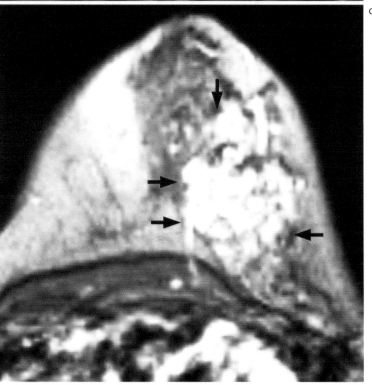

c

Fig. 58

Indications

Figs 58a–d
Asymmetric and irregular
breast tissue.
The patient was referred to
MRI because of the asymmetric and mammographically
quite irregular-appearing
tissue in the upper outer
quadrant combined with a
slight palpable abnormality.

a) Mammogram, craniocaudad view.

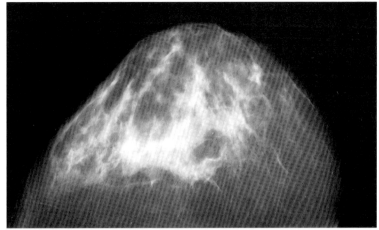

b) Mammogram, mediolateral
view.

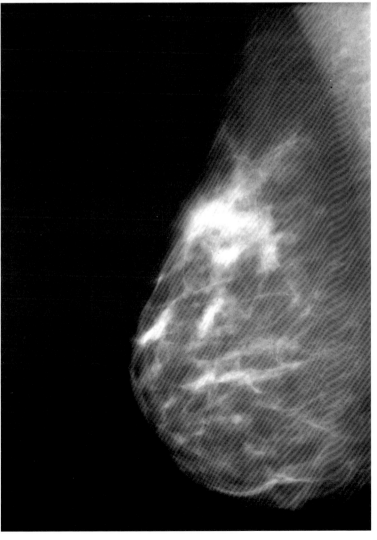

Fig. 58

c) Precontrast MR image, representative slice through the irregular tissue (from 32 slices of a FLASH 3D study: TR = 40 ms, TE = 14 ms, FA = 50°).

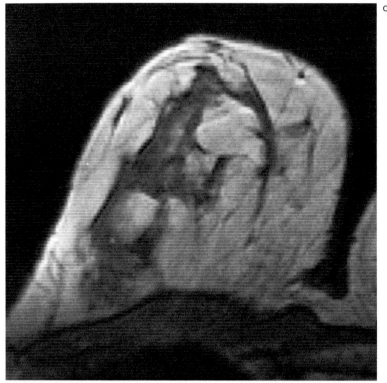

c

d) Postcontrast MR image. Malignancy was excluded based on absence of enhancement. Thus, close follow-up was recommended instead of biopsy.

Diagnosis: asymmetric breast tissue, confirmed by further follow-up (1½ years).

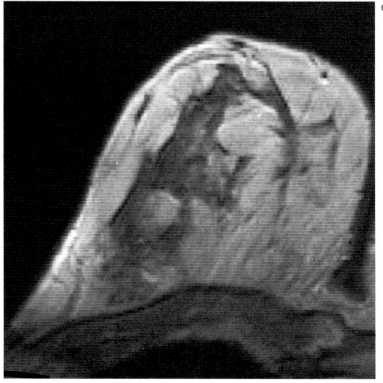

d

Fig. 59

Indications

Figs. 59a–d
Asymmetric tissue.
This patient was referred to
MRI because of a moderate
palpable asymmetry com-
bined with mammographi-
cally asymmetric increased
density in the upper outer
quadrant containing diffuse
microcalcifications.

a) Mammogram, cranio-
caudad view.

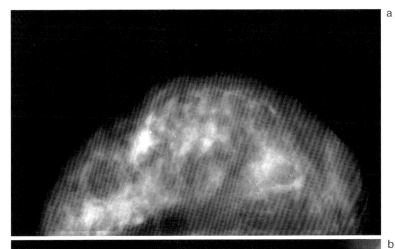

a

b) Mammogram, mediolateral
view.

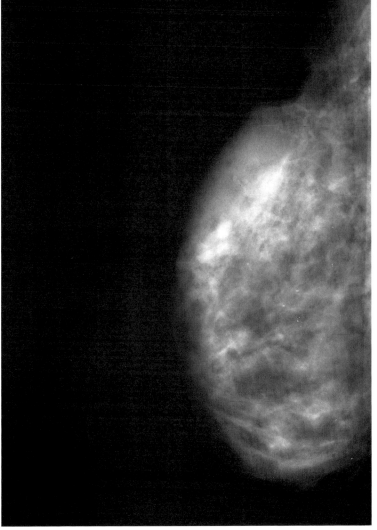

b

Fig. 59

c) Precontrast MR image at the level of the palpable asymmetry (representative slice of 32 images of a FLASH 3D study: TR = 40 ms, TE = 14 ms, FA = 50°).

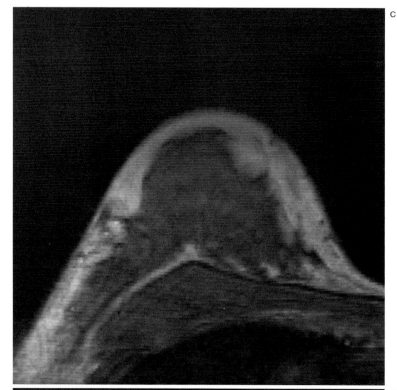

c

d) Postcontrast MR image (same slice, same pulse sequence) shows strong diffuse enhancement within the complete breast tissue including the area in question. Even though these findings are compatible with proliferative dysplasia, malignancy cannot be excluded.

Therefore, MRI was not helpful in this case and biopsy remained necessary for further classification of the palpable and mammographic findings.

Histology: proliferative dysplasia.

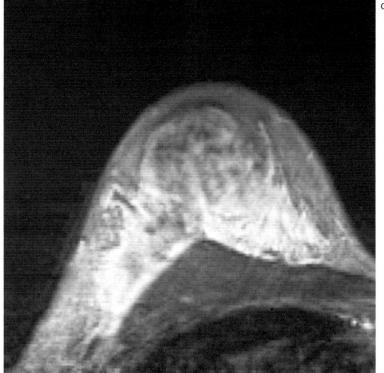

d

Fig. 60

Indications

Figs. 60a–c
Irregular, asymmetric density. The patient presented with an asymmetric irregular density of unknown etiology in the upper inner quadrant on the baseline mammogram. No palpable abnormality.

a) Right and left mammograms, mediolateral views.

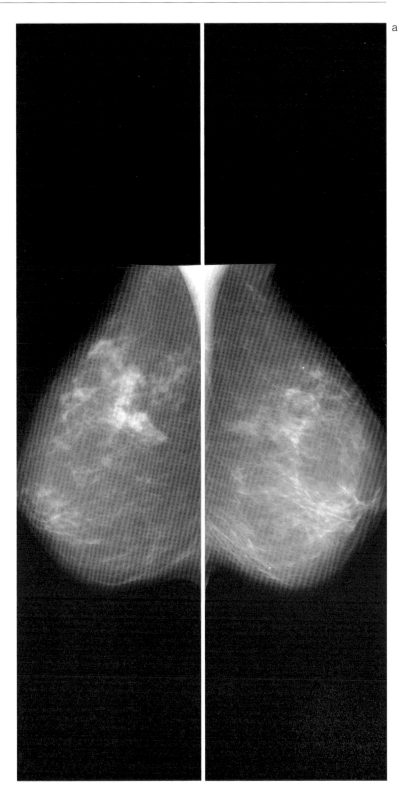

a

Fig. 60

b) Precontrast MR image at the level of the asymmetric density (one of 32 images of a FLASH 3D study: TR = 40 ms, TE = 14 ms, FA = 50°).

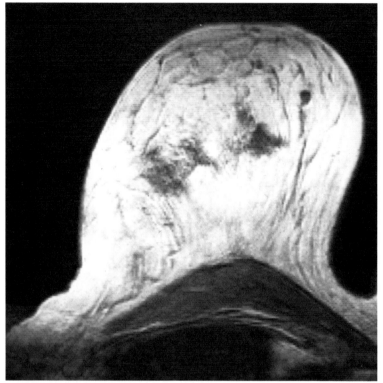

b

c) Postcontrast MR image (same slice, same pulse sequence). Because of the absent enhancement within the asymmetric tissue, malignancy could be excluded and close follow-up was recommended instead of biopsy.

Diagnosis: asymmetric tissue, confirmed by 2-year follow-up.

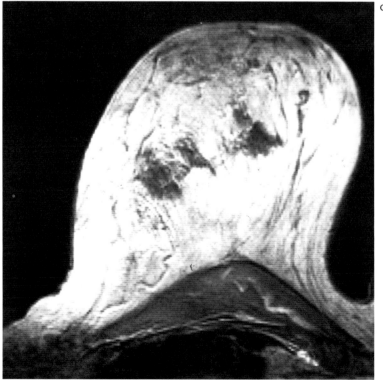

c

Fig. 61   Indications

Figs. 61a–c
Another patient with an irregular asymmetric density. This patient, too, presented with asymmetric irregular density on the baseline mammogram of her right breast.
There was no definite palpable abnormality within the large breast.

a) Right and left mammogram, mediolateral views.

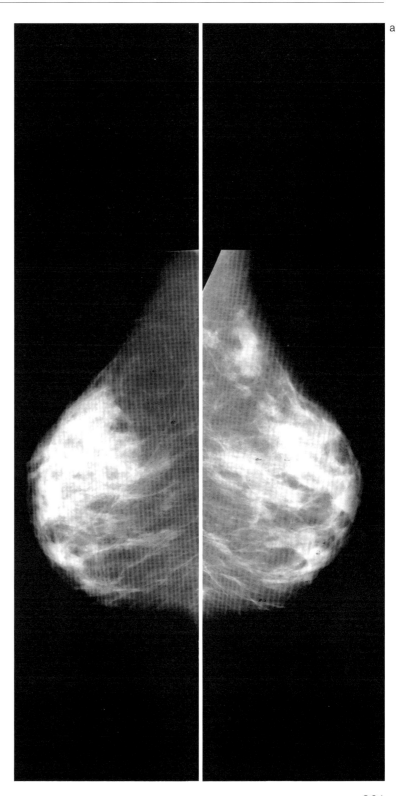

a

Fig. 61

b) Precontrast MR image at the level of the irregular tissue (FLASH 2D: TR = 30 ms, TE = 13 ms, FA = 50°).

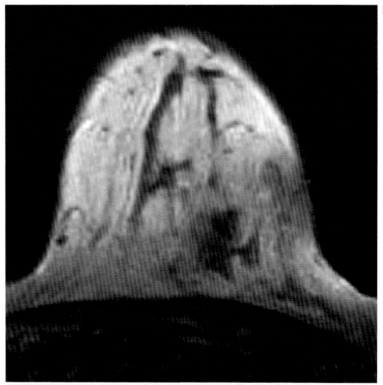

c) Postcontrast MR image (same slice, same pulse sequence) demonstrates the irregular tissue, which does not enhance significantly. In the center of this area, however, a smaller lesion with significant enhancement (arrows) is visualized. Differential diagnosis: benign or malignant tumor. Therefore, biopsy was recommended.

Histology: dysplasia containing a small fibroadenoma.

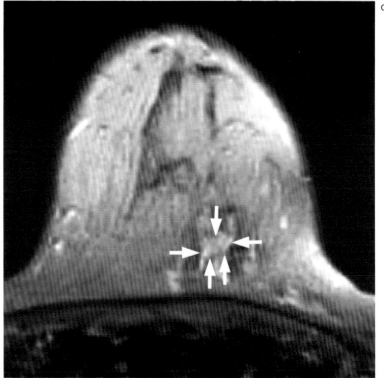

Fig. 62

Indications

Figs. 62a–d
Mammographic irregular density visible on two of three views.
This patient presented with a mammographically detected starlike density visible on the mediolateral and oblique views. MRI was requested for better characterization and, if necessary, for exact localization. There was no palpable abnormality.

a) Mammogram, oblique view, which shows the suspicious density.

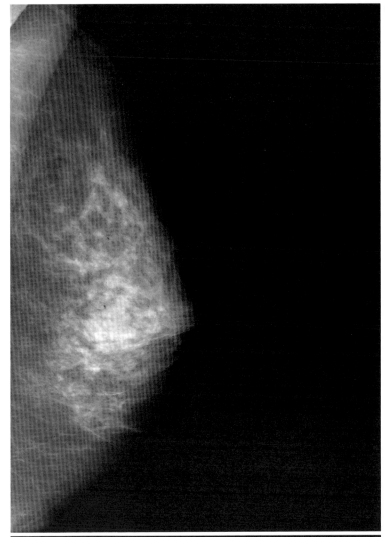

a

b) Mammogram, craniocaudad view. On this view it was not possible to localize the lesion.

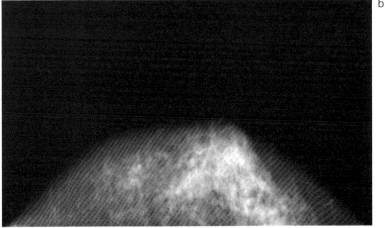

b

Fig. 62

c) Representative precontrast MR image of the upper quadrants (one of 32 slices, FLASH 3D: TR = 40 ms, TE = 14 ms, FA = 50°).

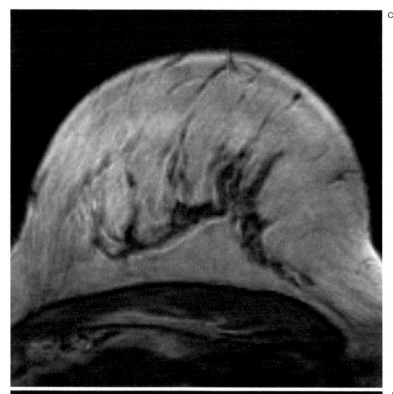

c

d) Postcontrast MR image (same slice, same pulse sequence). No definite mass is visible on the tomographic MR images (slice thickness 4 mm). Based on the non-significant enhancement of the complete breast tissue, malignancy was exluded by MRI.

Diagnosis: nodular dysplasia and superimposition, confirmed by follow-up (>1 year).

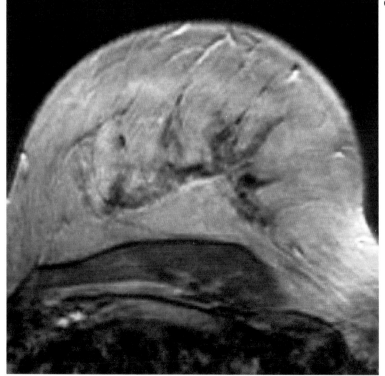

d

Fig. 63   Indications

Figs. 63a–d
Slight retraction of the skin
without palpable mass in the
medial inframammary fold of
unknown etiology.
The patient was referred to
MRI for further evaluation,
since a definite abnormality
could not be detected sonographically or mammographically using multiple views.

a) Mammogram, oblique view.

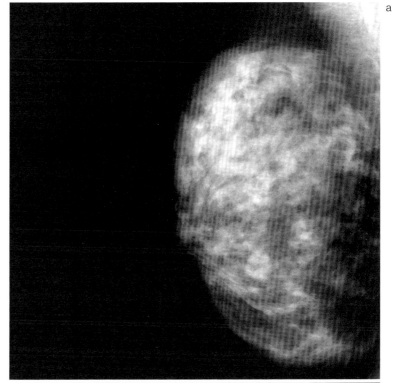

a

b) Mammogram, special view
with markers in the questionable area and on the nipple.
(Figs. a and b with kind permission from Dr. J. R. Hüppe
and Dr. H.-J. Schneider,
Munich).

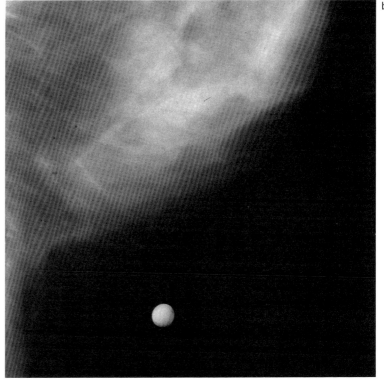

b

Fig. 63

c) Precontrast MR image at the level of the slight retraction (one of 32 images of a FLASH 3D study: TR = 40 ms, TE = 14 ms, FA = 50°).

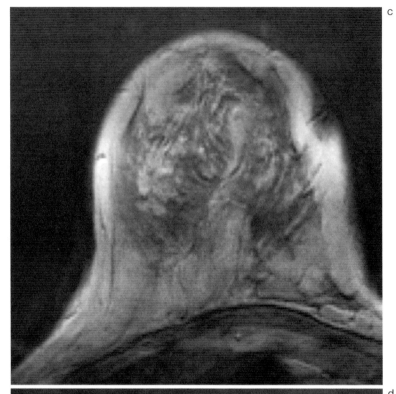

c

d) Postcontrast MR image (same slice, same pulse sequence) exhibits significant enhancement in a small area above the inframammary fold (arrow). Based on this enhancement, biopsy was strongly recommended.

Histology: T1 ductal and intraductal carcinoma.

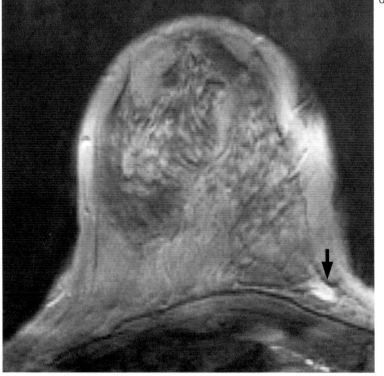

d

Fig. 64   Indications

Figs. 64a–f
Mammographically suspicious irregular density, visible on one view only. The patient presented with no palpable abnormality, but with the irregular density (arrow), which was visible on one view of the baseline mammogram only. Sonography was inconclusive because of shadowing and the surrounding hypoechoic fat.

a) Mammogram, mediolateral view, showing an irregular density (arrow) below a fibrosed fibroadenoma with calcification (arrowhead).

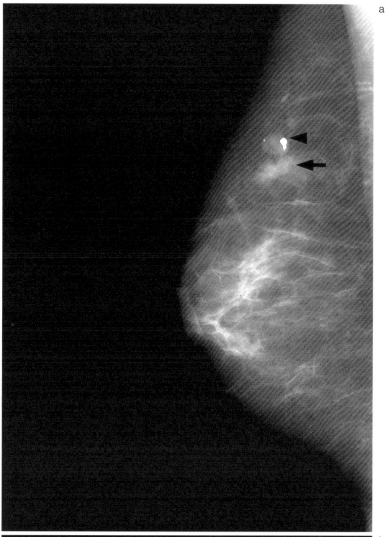

a

b) On further views, as on this craniocaudad mammographic view, the irregular lesion could not be exactly localized.

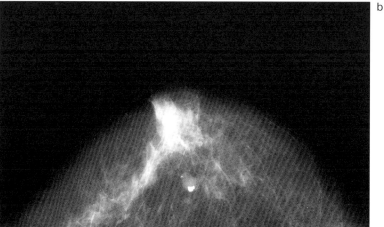

b

Fig. 64

c) Precontrast MR image at the level of the mammographic abnormality (FLASH 3D: TR = 40 ms, TE = 40 ms, FA = 50°).

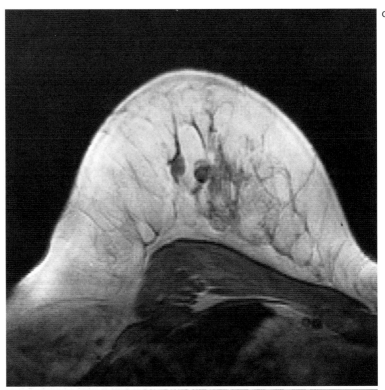

d) Postcontrast MR image (same slice, same pulse sequence) demonstrates two round lesions (arrow and arrowhead), as well as irregular tissue, which continues on the neighboring slice (e). None of the tissue shown enhances.

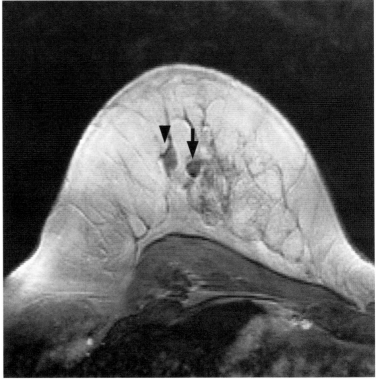

Fig. 64   Indications

e, f) Pre- and postcontrast MR images of the neighboring slice (same pulse sequence) demonstrates the nonenhancing irregular tissue.

Based on the MRI findings, the mammographically suspicious density can be explained as superimposition of irregularly shaped dysplasia (arrow) and a second fibroadenoma (see arrow Fig. 64 d), which on MRI with the patient in the prone position is located medially to the first calcified fibroadenoma (arrowhead). Due to nonsignificant enhancement within the complete breast, malignancy was excluded.

Diagnosis: superimposition of fibroadenoma and dysplasia, confirmed by 1-year follow-up.

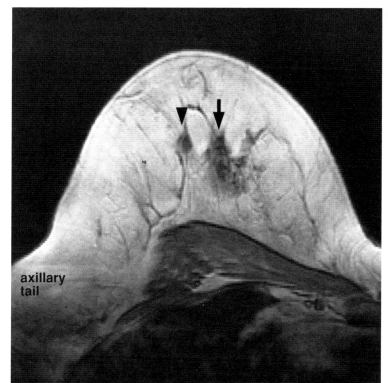

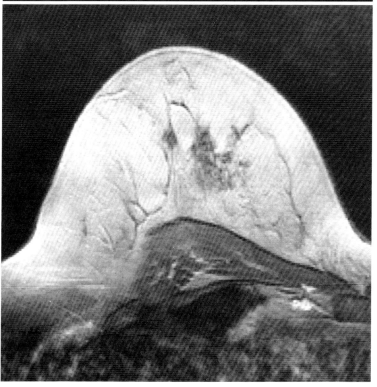

Fig. 65

Figs. 65a–f a
Starlike density of unknown etiology visible on one view only in a patient with known scarring.

a) Mammogram mediolateral view 1986.

b) Mammogram mediolateral view 1988.

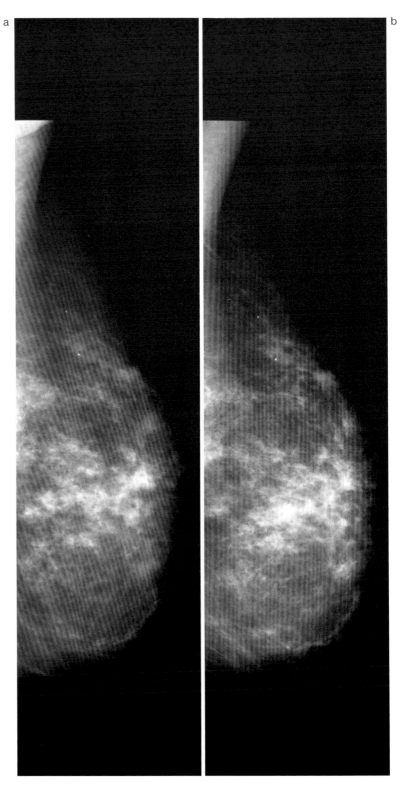

Fig. 65   Indications

c) Mammogram, cranio-
caudad view 1986.

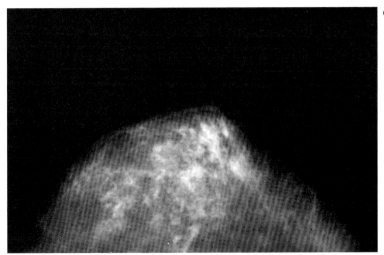

d) Mammogram, cranio-
caudad view 1988.

The patient presented with no
palpable abnormality. Several
starlike nodules caused by
scarring after excision of a
fibroadenoma were known
(a, c). On the mediolateral
mammograms no significant
change was noted compared
to 2 years before (a, b).
However, on the craniocaudad view a faint starlike
lesion had newly appeared
(c, d). Since it could not be
associated with a new lesion
on the mediolateral view, an
MRI study was performed to
exclude superimposition, to
evaluate the benignity of this
finding (differential diagnosis: starlike scarring in a
different projection), and
possibly to locate it.

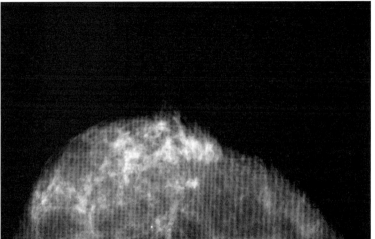

Fig. 65

e) Precontrast MR image through the upper part of the patient's breast (one of 32 slices of a FLASH 3D study: TR = 40 ms, TE = 14 ms, FA = 50°).

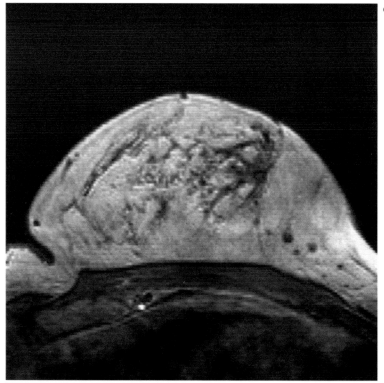

e

f) Postcontrast image (same slice, same pulse sequence) demonstrates a tiny irregular enhancing lesion (arrow), compatible with the mammographic finding on the craniocaudad view.

Because of the significant enhancement, biopsy was recommended and performed after MR-guided needle localization.

Histology confirmed a 5-mm ductal carcinoma.

from (50)

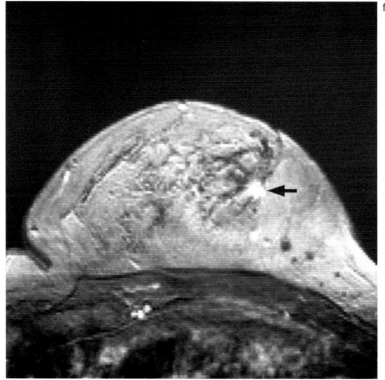

f

Fig. 66

Indications

Figs. 66a–f a
Irregular scarring with questionable increased density on one view only.
The patient, status post excision of a lobular carcinoma in situ several years ago, presented with a starlike questionably increased density predominantly visible on the mediolateral view (arrow). Due to thickening within the scar and diffuse shadowing, both palpation and sonography were inconclusive.

a) Mediolateral mammogram one year before.

b) Mediolateral mammogram at presentation.

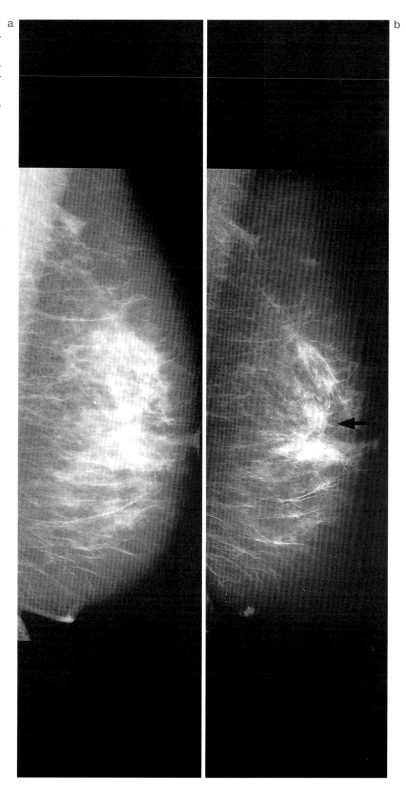

b

Fig. 66

c) Craniocaudad mammogram one year before.

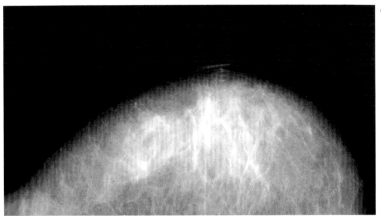

c

d) Craniocaudad mammogram at presentation.

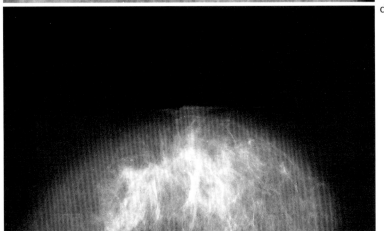

d

Fig. 66

Indications

e) Precontrast MR image (representative slice of 32 slices of a FLASH 3D study: TR = 40 ms, TE = 14 ms, FA = 50°).

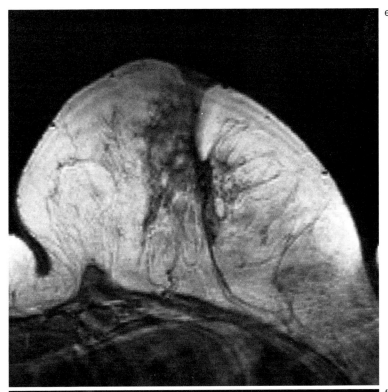

f) Postcontrast MR image (same slice, same pulse sequence).
On the tomographic MR images, no definite mass was visualized. Based on absence of significant enhancement within the irregular-appearing tissue (arrow), malignancy was excluded.

Diagnosis: scarring and varying superimposition, confirmed by 2-year follow-up.

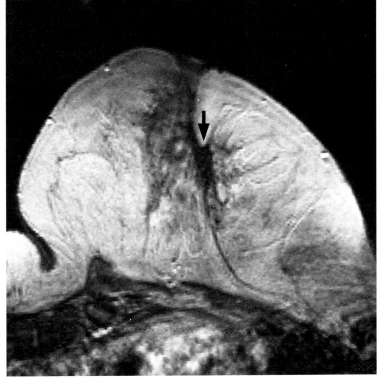

Fig. 67

Figs. 67a–e
Scarring and questionable palpable abnormality. The patient presented status post tumorectomy and radiation therapy 4 years ago with significant scarring and questionable palpable thickening within the scar. Since it could not be determined whether the palpable findings had changed or not, and since malignancy could not be excluded mammographically (due to dense tissue) or sonographically (due to multiple hypoechoic areas) MRI was recommended.

a) Mammogram, craniocaudad view.

b) Mammogram, mediolateral view.

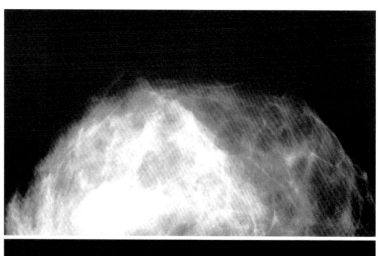
a

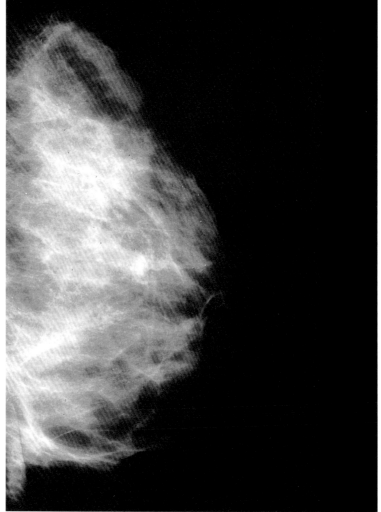
b

Fig. 67

Indications

c) Precontrast MR image (one of 32 slices of a FLASH 3D study: TR = 40 ms, TE = 14 ms, FA = 50°) at the level of the scar and the palpable findings.

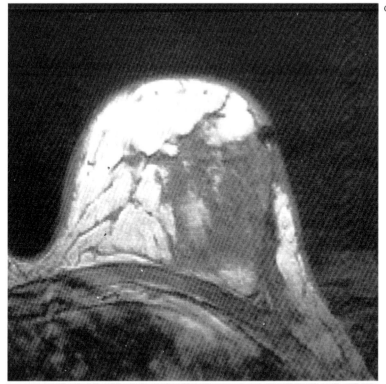

c

d) Postcontrast MR image (same slice, same pulse sequence) exhibits no enhancement at all. The signal void and skin thickening indicate scarring.

Based on these findings, malignancy was excluded and follow-up recommended instead of biopsy.

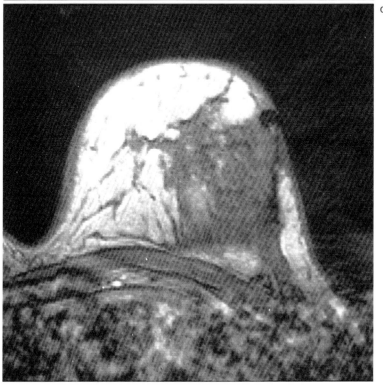

d

Fig. 67

e) Sonogram.

Diagnosis: scarring, con-
firmed by 2-year follow-up.

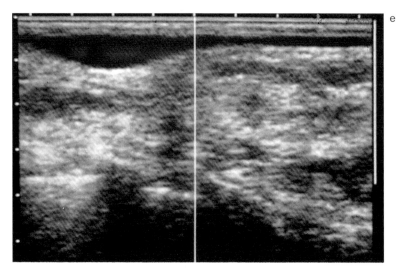

e

Fig. 68

Indications

Figs. 68a–e
Exclusion of further malignancy.
The patient was referred for
MRI 3 weeks after biopsy of a
fibroadenoma at 12 o'clock at
the upper margin of the
breast. Histologically by
chance a small carcinoma
had been detected directly
adjacent to the fibroadenoma.
Since neither the fibroadenoma nor the carcinoma had
been visible on the prebiopsy
mammograms, MRI was
desired for exclusion of
further carcinomatous tissue
before the planned excision
of the previous biopsy site.
Clinical examination and
sonography, performed
before MRI, were normal.
The MR images at the biopsy
site (not shown here) exhibited slight delayed en-
hancement, compatible with
status post surgery. Exclusion of microscopic remaining tumor is, of course, not
possible by MRI and was not
desired.

a) Outside mammogram,
craniocaudad view
before biopsy.

b) Outside mammogram,
mediolateral view
before biopsy.

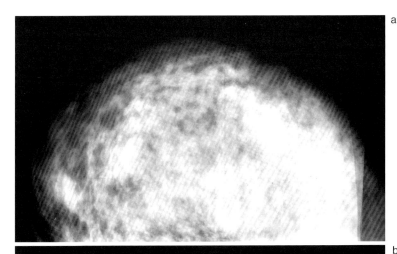

a

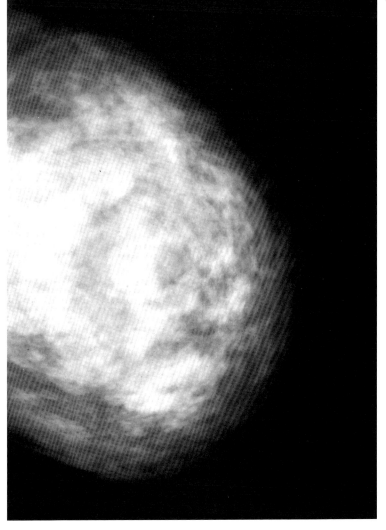

b

Fig. 68

c) Precontrast image at the center of the breast far away from the initial biopsy site (one of 32 slices of a FLASH 3D sequence: TR = 40 ms, TE = 14 ms, FA = 50°).

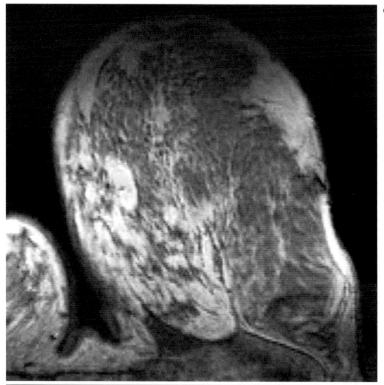

c

d) Postcontrast MR image (same slice, same pulse sequence), however, demonstrated a tiny enhancing lesion (arrow).

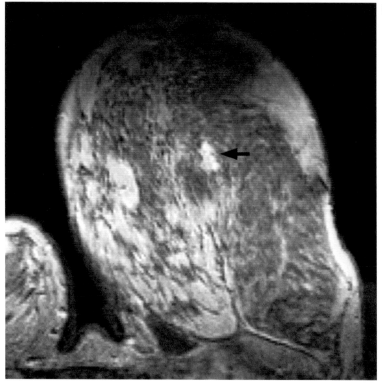

d

Fig. 68

Indications

e) The tiny suspicious lesion is even better visualized on the subtraction image (resulting from image d minus image c), which displays enhancing tissues such as the carcinoma and vessels only.

Since the tiny suspicious lesion was nonpalpable and since it was visualized by MRI alone, it was excised after MR-guided needle biopsy, performed simultaneously with excision of the previous biopsy site.

Histology: no further malignancy was detected at the initial biopsy site (not shown here). The tiny lesion (d, e) proved to be a small intraductal carcinoma.

from (50)

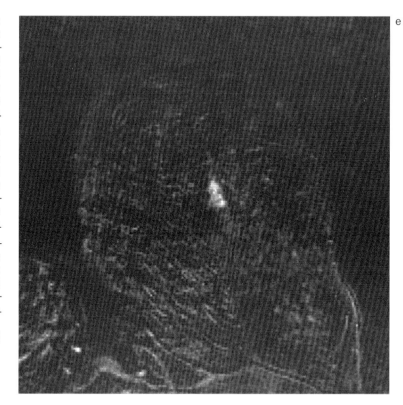

e

Fig. 69

Figs. 69a–d
Search for primary tumor. This patient presented without palpable abnormality after excision of axillary lymph nodes involved by adenocarcinoma of unknown origin. Mammographically, exclusion of malignancy appeared uncertain because of multiple nodular densities. Sonography was inconclusive due to multiple interposed fat lobules.

a) Mammogram, craniocaudad view.

b) Mammogram, mediolateral view.

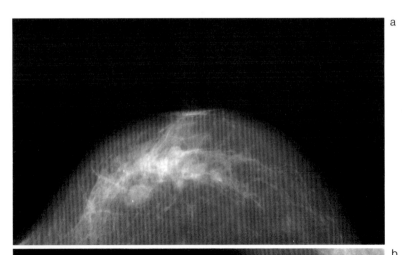

a

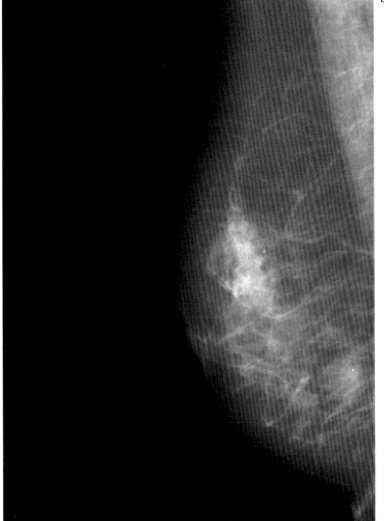

b

Fig. 69

Indications

c) Precontrast MR image (representative slice of 32 images of a FLASH 3D study: TR = 40 ms, TE = 14 ms, FA = 50°).

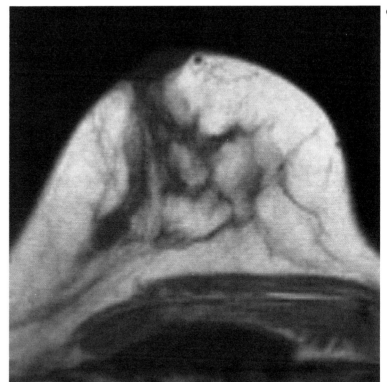

c

d) Postcontrast MR image (same slice, same pulse sequence) shows no significant enhancement within the breast tissue. The small nodules can be explained as nonenhancing cysts or nonenhancing completely fibrosed fibroadenomas (those nodules that were not anechoic sonographically). Based on the MRI study, malignancy within this breast was excluded.

Diagnosis: no sign of malignancy within the breast, confirmed by 2-year follow-up.

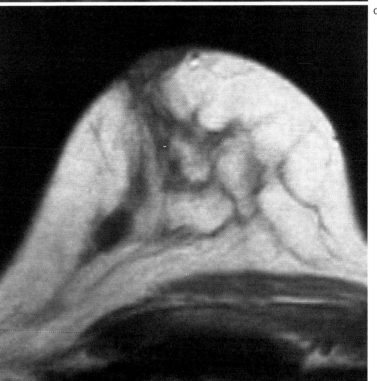

d

Fig. 70

Figs. 70a–d
Search for malignancy. The patient presented status post contralateral mastectomy and reconstructive surgery because of breast carcinoma, with a newly enlarged lymph node in the right axilla.
MRI of the right breast was recommended, since malignancy could neither be excluded clinically within the large nodular breast tissue nor mammographically because of the very dense tissue.

a) Craniocaudad mammogram.

b) Mediolateral mammogram.
(Figs. a and b with kind permission from Dr. J. R. Hüppe and Dr. H.-J. Schneider, Munich)

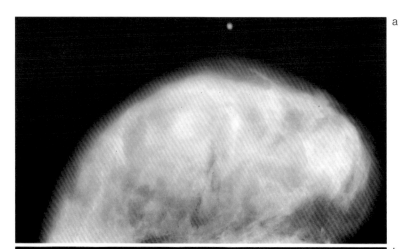

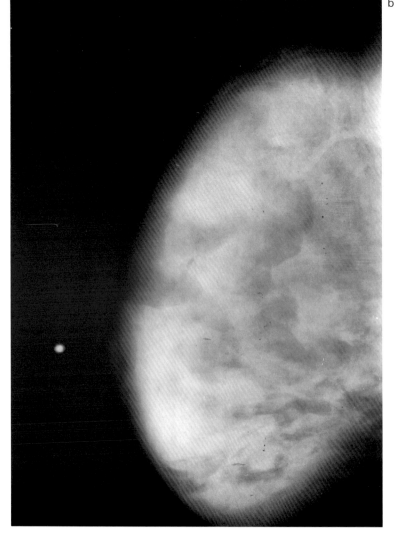

Fig. 70

Indications

c) Precontrast MR image (representative slice of 32 images of a FLASH 3D study) through the center of the right breast.

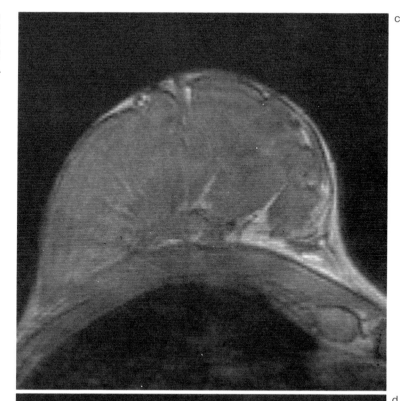

c

d) Postcontrast MR image (same slice, same pulse sequence) exhibits patchy significant enhancement within the complete breast tissue. In addition, an oval, strongly and fast-enhancing lesion (arrow) was detected centrally close to the pectoral muscle. Based on the history, the enlarged lymph node, and the MRI appearance biopsy of this suspicious lesion was recommended. Unfortunately, because of the diffuse and patchy enhancement, malignancy could not be excluded by MRI in the remaining tissue.

Because of the generally very difficult evaluation and the patient's history, subcutaneous mastectomy was performed.

Histology: the strongly enhancing lesion proved to be a fibroadenoma. The remaining tissue consisted of proliferative dysplasia. The lymph node exhibited inflammatory changes.

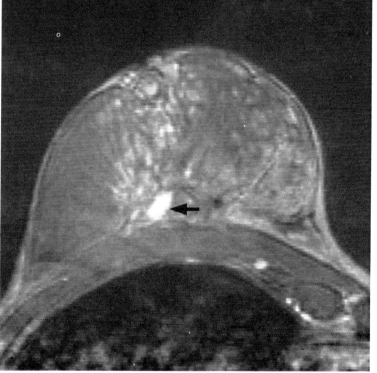

d

Fig. 71

Figs. 71a–d
Search for primary tumor.
This patient was referred to
MRI after excision of axillary
lymph nodes containing
adenocarcinoma of unknown
origin. No palpable abnormality was detected in either
breast.
Mammography, which was
somewhat impaired by the
very dense tissue, and sonography did not show a sign of
malignancy.

a) Mammogram, craniocaudad view.

b) Mammogram, mediolateral
view. (Figs. a and b with kind
permission from
Dr. J. R. Hüppe and
Dr. H.-J. Schneider, Munich)

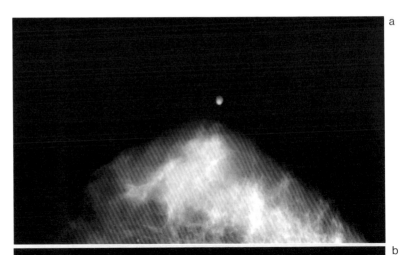

a

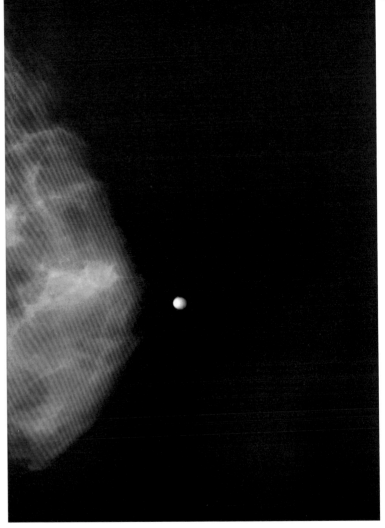

b

Fig. 71   Indications

c) Precontrast MR image at the center of the breast (one of 32 slices of FLASH 3D: TR = 40 ms, TE = 14 ms, FA = 50°).

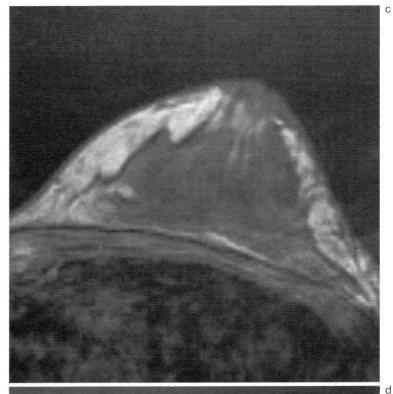

c

d) Postcontrast MR image (same slice, same pulse sequence) exhibits a strongly enhancing area medially in the breast . Since the abnormality was not palpable, even in retrospect, and was not shown by other modalities either, MR-guided biopsy had to be performed.

Histology: an intraductal carcinoma corresponding to the MR image was found, which contained a tiny invasive area of 4 mm.

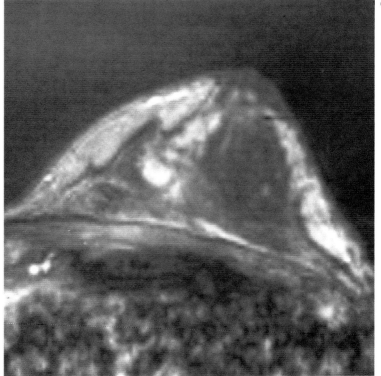

d

Fig. 72

Figs. 72a–e
Quiz:
Interesting case.
No history given. What do the
images show?

a) Craniocaudad mam-
mogram.

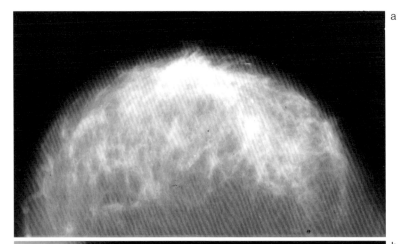

b) Mediolateral mammogram.

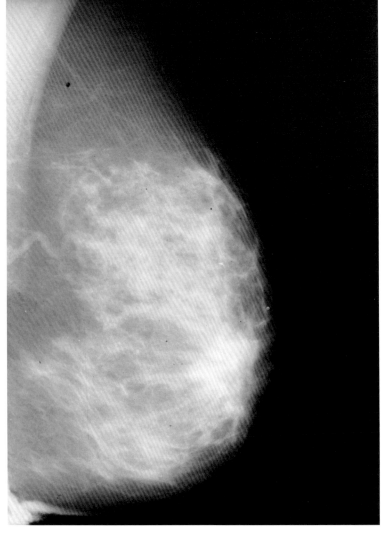

Answer this question before
you go on to the next page.

Answer:
A starlike lesion is visualized
behind the nipple.

Fig. 72

Quiz

Question:
Based on MRI, is this starlike
lesion probably benign (scarring) or malignant?

c) Precontrast MR image at
the level of the nipple (one of
32 slices of a FLASH 3D
study: TR = 40 ms,
TE = 14 ms, FA = 50°).

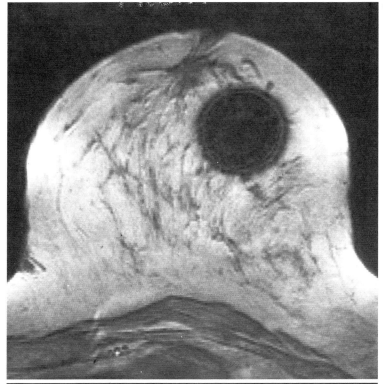

c

d) Postcontrast MR image
(same slice, same pulse
sequence).

Histology: ductal carcinoma.
Answer:
Because of its irregular
contours and its significant
enhancement the lesion is
highly suspicious.

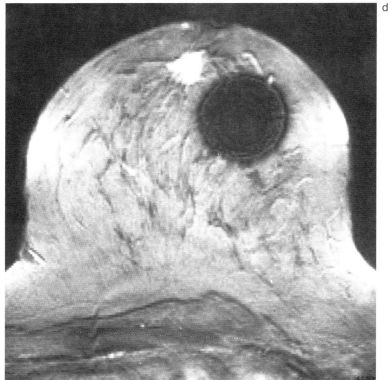

d

Question:
Can you explain the other
finding on the MR image?

Fig. 72

e) Magnified section of the craniocaudad mammogram.

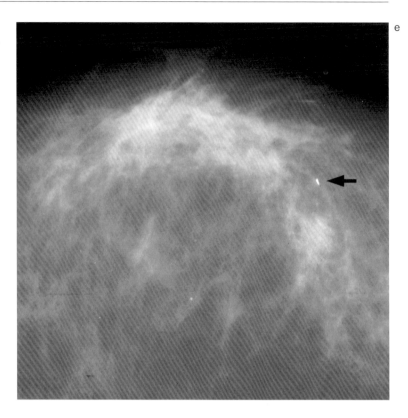

e

Answer:
The signal void is ideally round and unchanged on pre- and postcontrast scans.

This feature is typical for a metal artifact. Analyzing the mammogram more closely, you can recognize a tiny metal piece (arrow) (a, e), probably a tiny piece of needle from a biopsy several years before.
Note also the significant change of position between the tumor and the metal piece when comparing the mammogram, obtained in the upright position, and the MR images acquired in the prone position.

Present state and future aspect

Contrast-enhanced MRI of the breast is still a relatively young discipline and consequently not yet widely used, partly because Gd-DTPA and breast coils are not yet readily available.

Nevertheless future possibilities of contrast-enhanced MRI should not be underestimated: Although the percentage of diagnostically difficult cases, in which decision between biopsy or follow-up is especially problematic with conventional methods, is low in relative terms, the absolute number of cases is still high. With increased use of mammographic screening, the number of very small and therefore uncharacteristic lesions will rise further. On the one hand, unnecessary biopsy (indicated by high biopsy rates) leads to increased scarring, further diagnostic problems, and decreasing confidence in the diagnostic methods (14). On the other hand, delayed diagnosis (caused by too long follow-up) must also be avoided. Therefore, an additional tool like contrast-enhanced MRI appears very helpful. Contrast-enhanced MRI has so far proven able to exclude or detect malignancy in complicated cases, thus helping to avoid unnecessary biopsies and improve accuracy.

Because contrast-enhanced MRI of the breast is so young, further confirmation of the present results in well-designed studies with regular follow-up is desirable.

Future technical optimizations should include the following:

– Further shortening of acquisition and imaging time.

– Further reduction of artifacts, especially motion artifacts of the heart.

– Further optimization of coil design (especially of the double breast coil, see page 24).

– Development and investigation of further pulse sequences.

It might be interesting to investigate other MRI contrast media as well (high-molecular components of Gd-DTPA, nonionic MRI contrast media, and compounds, including specific antibodies or certain porphyrin derivates) to improve specificity of enhancing lesions (123).

In summary, contrast-enhanced MRI of the breast has already proven a very interesting method, which may provide precious additional information. Nevertheless, further development and improvements are still desirable and possible.

References

1. D'Agincourt L
Advances in mammography improve cancer detection
Diagnostic imaging (1989) 90–98

2. Alcorn FS, Turner DA, Clark JW et al
Magnetic resonance imaging in the study of the breast
Radiographics (1985) 5:631–652

3. American College of Radiology
College policy reviews use of thermography
Amer Coll Radiol Bull (1984) 40:13

4. Axel L
Surface coil MRI
J Comput Assist Tomogr (1984) 8:381–384

5. Bässler R
Pathologie der Brustdrüse
Berlin, Heidelberg, New York: Springer 1978
Spez pathol Anatomie, Bd 11

6. Bässler R, Kreienberg R, Scheidt E
Ergebnisse pathologischer und differentialdiagnostischer Untersuchungen an 4000 Probeexcisionen der Mamma
Arch Gynäk (1972) 211:48

7. Baker LH
BCDDP
Five year summary report
Cancer 1982; 32/4:194–225

8. Barth V
Röntgen wie? wann? – Brustdrüse
Stuttgart: Thieme 1979

9. Barth V, Prechtel K
Atlas der Brustdrüse und ihrer Erkrankungen
Stuttgart: Enke 1990

10. Bassett LW, Gold RH
Mammography, thermography and ultrasound in breast cancer detection
New York, London: Grune & Stratton 1982

11. Bassett LW, Kimme-Smith C, Sutherland LK et al
Automated and held breast ultrasound: effect on patient management
Radiology (1987) 165:103–108

12. Bibbo M, Schreiber M, Cajulis R et al
Stereotactic fine needle aspiration cytology of clinically occult malignant and premalignant breast lesions
Acta cytol (1988) 32:193–201

13. Bloomer WD, Berenberg AL, Weissman BN
Mammography of the definitively irradiated breast
Radiology (1976) 118:425–428

14. Brenner RJ, Sickles EA
Acceptability of periodic follow-up as an alternative to biopsy for mammographically detected lesions interpreted as probably benign
Radiology (1989) 171:645–646

15. Bydder GM, Curati WL, Gadian DG et al
Use of closely coupled receiver coils in MRI: practical aspects
J Comput Assist Tomogr (1985) 9/5:987–996

16. Chacko AK, Tottermann S, Rubens D et al
Paramagnetic enhancement accentuation by chemical shift imaging in the breast: improvement in lesion visualisation
Radiology (1989) 173(P):354

17. Cole-Beuglet C, Schwartz G, Kurtz B et al
Ultrasound mammography for the augmented breast
Radiology (1983) 146:737–742

18. Damadian R, Zaner K, Hor D et al
Tumors by NMR
Physiol Chem Phys (1973) 5:381–402

19. Deimling M, Loeffler W
Fast simultaneous acquisition of fat and water images
Book of Abstracts 8th Annual Meeting
Amsterdam: Soc Magn Res in Med (1989) 837

20. Deimling M, Sauter R, König H et al
Fast chemical shift imaging: application on 3D acquisition
Book of abstracts, 6th Annual Meeting
New York: Soc Magn Res in Med (1987) 447

21. Dershaw DD, Chaglassian TA
Mammography after prothesis placement for augmentation or reconstructive mammoplasty
Radiology (1989) 170:69–74

22. Egger H, Weishaar J, Hamperl H
Sterne im Mammogramm – Karzinome und strahlige Narben
Geburtsh Frauenheilk (1976) 36:547–553

23. El Yousef SJ, Duchesneau RH, Alfidi RJ et al
Magnetic resonance imaging of the breast
Radiology (1984) 150:761–766

24. El Yousef SJ, O'Connell DM, Duchesneau RH et al
Benign and malignant breast disease: magnetic resonance and radiofrequency pulse sequences
Amer J Roentgenol (1985) 145:1–8

25. Feig SA
Decreased breast cancer mortality through mammographic screening: results of clinical trials
Radiology (1988) 167:659–665

26. Feig SA
Benefits and risks of mammography
in: Brünner S, Langfeldt B, Anderson PE (eds)
Early detection of breast cancer
Berlin, Heidelberg, New York: Springer 1984

27. Flamm MB
Breast masses: US-guided fine-needle aspiration biopsy. Letter to the Editor
Radiology (1987) 163:831

28. Fornage BD, Lorigan JG, Andry E
Fibroadenoma of the breast: sonographic appearance
Radiology (1989) 172:671–675

29. Gad A, Thomas A, Moskowitz M
Screening for breast cancer in Europe. Achievements, problems, and future
in: Brünner S, Langfeldt B, Anderson PE (eds)
Early detection of breast cancer
Berlin, Heidelberg, New York: Springer 1984

30. Gersonde K, Staemmler M, Felsberg L
Gewebecharakterisierung durch parameterselektive Kernspintomographie. Identifizierung von weiblichen Brusttumoren.
in: Lissner J, Doppman JL, Margulis AR (eds)
MR'87
Konstanz: Schnetztor 1988, 365–367

31. Gisvold JJ, Brown LR, Swee RG et al
Comparison of mammography and transillumination light scanning in the detection of breast lesions
Amer J Roentgenol (1986) 147/1:191-194

32. Gohagan JK, Spitznagel EL, Murphy WA et al
Multispectral analysis of MR images of the breast
Radiology (1987) 163:703–707

33. Gordenne WH, Malchair FL
Mach bands in mammography
Radiology (1988) 169:55–58

34. Hackeloer BJ, Duda V, Lauth G
Ultraschall-Mammographie: Methoden, Ergebnisse, diagnostische Strategien
Berlin, Heidelberg, New York: Springer 1986

35. Hayes H, Vandergift J, Diner WC
Mammography and breast implants
Plast Reconstr Surg (1988) 82:1–8

36. Hermann G, Keller RJ, Schwartz J et al
Non-palpable breast masses: radiologic predictability of malignancy
Radiology (1988) 169(P):60

37. Hermansen C, Skovgaard Poulsen H, Langfeldt B et al
Diagnostic reliability of combined physical examination, mammography and fine-needle puncture (triple–test) in breast tumors
Cancer (1987) 60(8):1866–1871

38. Heywang SH
Contrast-enhanced MRI of the breast
in: Runge VM (ed)
Enhanced magnetic resonance imaging
St Louis: Mosby 1988 (232–243)

38a. Heywang SH
MRI does not replace mammography-present state of MRI of the breast with and without contrast agent
J Med Imaging (1988) 8:817–826

39. Heywang SH
Contrast-enhanced MRI of the breast using Gd-DTPA
Diagn Imaging Internat (1988) (suppl): 34–36

39a. Heywang SH, Hilbertz T, Pruss E
MR-Diagnostik und Gd-DTPA und schnelle Sequenzen bei Erkrankungen der Mamma
Der Nuklearmediziner (1988) 4:221–229

40. Heywang SH
KM-verstärkte MRT der Mamma
in: Bydder GM et al (eds)
Contrast media in MRI
Proceedings of the international workshop
Berlin: Medicom Europe 1990 (in press)

41. Heywang SH, Beck R, Hilbertz T et al
MR imaging with Gd-DTPA in the breast after limited surgery and radiation therapy
Radiology (1989) 173(P):230

42. Heywang SH, Hilbertz T, Beck R et al
MR-gestützte Lokalisation kernspintomographisch suspekter Mammabefunde
Zentralbl Radiol (1990) 141/3–4:215

43. Heywang SH, Deimling M, Hilbertz T et al
Improved sequences for T1 and T2 quantification: first applications in breast imaging
Radiology (1988) 169(P):326

44. Heywang SH, Dritschilo A, Cigtay O
Erste Erfahrungen bei der mammographischen Rezidiverkennung nach Tylektomie und Bestrahlung
Fortschr Roentgenstr (1984) 141/4:438–441

44a. Heywang SH, Eiermann W, Bassermann R et al
Carcinoma of the breast behind a prosthesis – comparison of ultrasound, mammography and MRI
Comput Radiol (1985) 9:283–286

45. Heywang SH, Fenzl G, Baierl P et al
Differential diagnosis of breast masses by MRI
Proceedings, 4th Annual Meeting
London: Soc Magn Res in Med (1985) 1154

46. Heywang SH, Fenzl G, Beck R et al
Anwendung von Gd-DTPA bei der kernspintomographischen Untersuchung der Mamma
Fortschr Roentgenstr (1986) 145/5:565–571

47. Heywang SH, Fenzl G, Hahn D et al
MR of the breast: histopathologic correlation
Eur J Radiol (1987) 3/7:175–183

48. Heywang SH, Hahn D, Schmid H et al
MR imaging of the breast using Gadolinium-DTPA
J Comput Assist Tomogr (1986) 10:199–204

49. Heywang SH, Hilbertz T, Bauer WM et al
Kontrastmittel-Kernspintomographie der Mamma bei diagnostisch schwierigen Fällen
in: Lissner J, Doppman JL, Margulis AR (eds)
MR '89
Köln: Deutscher Ärzteverlag 1989, 138–142

50. Heywang SH, Hilbertz T, Beck R et al
Contrast-material enhanced MRI of the breast in patients with post-operative scarring and silicon implants
J Comput Assist Tomogr (1990) 14/3:348–356

51. Heywang SH, Hilbertz T, Fenzl G
Mamma
in: Lissner J, Seiderer M (eds)
Klinische Kernspintomographie,
2. Aufl Stuttgart: Enke 1990,
445:481

52. Heywang SH, Hilbertz T, Permanetter W et al
Contrast-enhanced MRI of carcinomas of the breast – histopathologic correlation
Proceedings, 2nd European Congress of NMR in Medicine and Biology, Berlin 1988, 169

53. Heywang SH, Hilbertz T, Pruss E et al
Dynamische Kontrastmitteluntersuchungen mit FLASH bei Kernspintomographie der Mamma
Digitale Bilddiagnostik (1988) 7–13

54. Heywang SH, Hilbertz T, Pruss E et al
Dynamic studies of contrast enhancement in MRI of the breast
Book of Abstracts, 7th Annual Meeting
San Francisco: Soc Magn Res in Med (1988) 684

55. Heywang SH, Lipsit ER, Glassman LM et al
Specificity of ultrasonography in the diagnosis of benign breast masses
J Ultrasound Med (1984) 3:453–461

56. Heywang SH, Lissner J
A carcinoma of the breast behind a prothesis – choice of imaging modality
Comput Radiol (1987) 11/4:209–211

57. Heywang SH, Wolf A, Pruss E et al
MRI of the breast with Gd-DTPA – use and limitations
Radiology (1989) 171:95–103

58. Heywang SH, Yousry T, Pruss E et al
Contrast-enhanced MRI of the breast – present state and future developments
in: Matsuura K, Katayama H, Iio M (eds)
Advance and future trends of contrast media
Tokyo 1987, 263–270

59. Hilbertz T, Heywang SH, Beck R et al
FLASH-3D-Imaging of the breast: comparison with standard SE-technique
Mag Reson Imag (1989) 7/suppl 1:192

60. Hoeffken W, Lanyi M
Mammography
Philadelphia, London, Toronto:
W. B. Saunders 1977

61. Hohenberg G, Wolf G, Schmid A
Problematik der radiologischen Mammadiagnostik nach brusterhaltenden Operationen und Radiatio
Röntgen Bl 2 (1986) 39,3:57–59

62. Homer MJ
Breast imaging: pitfalls, controversies and some practical thoughts
Radiol Clin North Amer (1985) 23/3:459–472

63. Homer MJ
Imaging features and management of characteristically benign and probably benign breast lesions
Radiol Clin North Amer (1987) 25:939–951

64. Hornak JP, Szumowsky J, Rubens D et al
Breast MR imaging with loopgap resonators
Radiology (1986) 161(3):832–834

65. Ikeda DM, Anderson J
Ductal carcinoma in situ: atypical mammographic appearances
Radiology (1989) 172:661–666

66. Kaiser WA
MR imaging of the breast: optimal imaging technique, results, limitation and histopathologic correlation
Radiology (1989) 173(P):230

67. Kaiser WA, Kess H
Prototyp – Doppelspule für die
Mamma-MR-Messung
Fortschr Roentgenstr (1989)
151/1:103–105

68. Kaiser WA, Mittelmaier O
Dynamic contrast-enhanced MRI of
the breast using a double breast
coil – an important step towards
routine MR-breast examinations
Book of Abstracts 8th Annual
Meeting
Amsterdam: Soc Magn Res in Med
(1989) 689

69. Kaiser WA, Oppelt A
Kernspintomographie der Mamma
mit Schnellbildverfahren (FISP und
FLASH)
in: Lissner J, Doppman JL,
Margulis AR (eds)
MR '87
Konstanz: Schnetztor 1988,
303–310

70. Kaiser WA, Zeitler E
MR imaging of the breast: fast
imaging sequences with and
without Gd-DTPA
Radiology (1989) 170:681–686

70a. Kashanian F, Goldstein HA,
Hugo F et al
Rapid injection of Magnevist®.
Book of abstracts
Ann Meeting Amer Soc Neuroradiol
(1989): 80

71. Kessler M, Igl W, Krauss B et al
Vergleich von Mammographie und
automatisierter Sonographie an
700 Patientinnen
Fortschr Roentgenstr (1983)
138:331

72. Kessler M, Heywang SH
Spezielle Mammadiagnostik
in: Lissner J, Fink U (eds) Radiologie II
3. Aufl Stuttgart: Enke 1990 (in
press)

73. König H, Gohagan JK, Laub G et
al
Improved MR breast images by
contrast optimization using artificial
intelligence
Radiology (1986) 161(P):27

74. Kopans DB
Nonmammographic breast imaging
techniques. Current status and
future developments
Radiol Clin North Amer (1987)
25/5:961–971

75. Krimmel K, Koebrunner G,
Heywang SH
Anpassung einer Mammaspule an
klinische Bedürfnisse an 1 Tesla
Digitale Bilddiagnostik (1986)
6/3:101–110

76. Lamarque JL, Rodiere MJ,
Prat X et al
Breast pathology in MRI
Eur J Radiol (1986) 6:42–47

77. Lanyi M
Diagnostik und Differentialdia-
gnostik der Mammaverkalkungen
2. Aufl, Berlin, Heidelberg,
New York: Springer 1989

78. Leucht W, Rabe DR
Lehratlas der Mammasonographie
Stuttgart, New York: Thieme 1989

79. Lewis Jones H, Whitehouse GH,
Leinster SJ
Gadolinium enhancement in
assessment of recurrent breast
carcinoma.
Book of Abstracts, 8th Annual
Meeting
Amsterdam: Soc Magn Res in Med
(1990) 690

80. Loflin T, Mueller PR, Simeone J F
et al
In vitro determination of the MR
relaxation characteristics of normal
and pathologic body fluids
Proceedings American Roentgen
Ray Society Meeting, Boston 1985,
28

81. Lufkin R, Teresi, Hanafee W
New needle for MR-guided aspiration cytology of the head and neck
Amer J Roentgenol (1987)
149:380–382

82. Lukas P
Weibliches Genital – Mamma –
Geburtshilfe – Diagnostik mit bild-
gebenden Verfahren
in: Willgeroth F, Breit A (eds)
Klinische Radiologie
Berlin, New York: Springer 1989

83. Mansfield P, Morris PG, Ordidge R et al
Carcinoma of the breast imaged by nuclear magnetic resonance (NMR)
Brit J Radiol (1979) 52:242–243

84. Marsteller LP, Paredes ES de
Outcome of well-defined masses on mammography: how often are they malignant?
Radiology (1989) 173(P):459

85. McCrea ES, Johnston C, Keramati B
Cystosarcoma phylloides
South Med J (1986) 79/5:543–547

86. McSweeney MB, Murphy CM
Whole breast sonography
Radiol Clin North Amer (1985) 23/1:157–167

87. McSweeney MB, Small WC, Cerny V et al
Magnetic resonance imaging in the diagnosis of breast disease: use of transverse relaxation times
Radiology (1984) 153:741–744

88. Merritt CRB, Bergson RB, Sullivan MA et al
Stereotaxic guidance for breast biopsy localisation and aspiration
Radiology (1989) 173(P):457

89. Meyer JE, Amin E, Lindfors KK et al
Medullary carcinoma of the breast: mammographic and US appearance
Radiology (1989) 170:79–82

90. Meyer JE, Silverman P, Gandbhir L
Fat necrosis of the breast
Arch Surg (1978) 113:801–805

91. Mitnick JS, Roses DF, Harris MN et al
Circumscribed intraductal carcinoma of the breast
Radiology (1989) 170:423–425

92. Monsees B, Destouet JM, Gersell D
Light scan evaluation of nonpalpable breast lesions
Radiology (1987) 163/2:467–470

93. Moskowitz M
Screening is not diagnosis
Radiology (1979) 133:265–268

94. Moskowitz M
The predictive value of certain mammography signs in screening for breast cancer
Cancer (1983) 51:1007–1011

95. Murphy WA, Gohagan JK
Breast
in: Stark DD, Bradley WG jun (eds)
Magnetic resonance imaging
St. Louis: CV Mosby 1987

95a. Niendorf HP, Dinger JC, Haustein J et al
Tolerance of Gd-DTPA: clinical experience
in: Bydder GM et al (eds)
Contrast media in MRI
Proceedings of the international workshop
Berlin: Medicom Europe 1990

96. Page DL, Winfield AC
The dense mammogram
Amer J Roentgenol (1986) 147:487–489

97. Partain CL, Kulkarni MV, Price RR et al
Magnetic resonance imaging of the breast: functional T1 and three-dimensional imaging
Cariovasc Intervent Radiol (1986) 8:292–299

98. Paulus DD, Libshitz HJ
Breast
in: Libshitz HJ (ed)
Diagnostic roentgenology of radiotherapy change
Baltimore: Williams and Wilkins 1979

99. Pietruszka M, Burnes L
Cystosarcoma phylloides: a clinico-pathologic analysis of 42 cases
Cancer (1978) 41:1974–83

100. Piontek RW, Kase KR
Radiation transmission study of silicon elastomer for mammary prosthesis
Radiology (1980) 136:505–507

101. Prechtel K, Gehm O
Morphologisch faßbare Vorstadien des Mammakarzinoms
Österr Z Onkol (1975a) 2:122

102. Prechtel K, Gehm O
Pathologie der Vor- und Frühstadien des Mammakarzinoms
Verh Deut Ges Pathol (1975b) 59:498

103. Rebner M, Pennes DR, Adler DD et al
Breast microcalcifications after lumpectomy and radiation therapy
Radiology (1989) 170:691–693

104. Ross RJ, Thompson JS, Kim K et al
Nuclear magnetic resonance imaging and evaluation of human breast tissue: preliminary clinical trials
Radiology (1982) 143:195–205

105. Schmid RA, Ridlen MS, Dowlatshahi K et al
Fine-needle cytology of breast lesions seen on mammograms
Radiology (1989) 173(P):173

106. Schnapf DJ, Dabb RW, Tiruchelvam V et al
MRI of the postmastectomy reconstructed breast
Magn Reson Imag (1989) 7/suppl 1:122

107. Schneider JA
Invasive pappillary breast carcinoma: mammographic and sonographic appearance
Radiology (1989) 171:377–379

108. Seidman H, Gelb SK, Silverberg E et al
Survival experience in the BCDDP
Cancer (1987) 37:258–290

109. Shapiro S, Venet W, Strax P et al
Current results of the breast cancer screening randomized trial: the Health Insurance Plan (HIP) of Greater New York Study
in: Day NE, Miller AB (eds)
Screening for breast cancer
Toronto: Hogrefe International (in press)

110. Shaw de Paredes E
Atlas of film-screen mammography
Baltimore, Munich: Urban & Schwarzenberg 1989

111. Sickles EA, Herzog KA
Intramammary scar tissue: a mimic of the mammographic appearance of carcinoma
Amer J Roentgenol (1980) 135:350–353

112. Silverstein MJ, Gamagami P, Colburn WJ et al
Non-palpable breast lesions: diagnosis with slightly overpenetrated screen-film mammography and hook wire-directed biopsy in 1014 cases
Radiology (1989) 171:633–638

113. Stack J, Redmond V, Codd MB et al
Tissue enhancement profiles with Gd-DTPA in breast carcinoma
Radiology (1988) 169(P):22

114. Stefanik DF, Brereton HD, Lee TC et al
Fat necrosis following breast irradiation for carcinoma: clinical presentation and diagnosis
Breast (1982) 8:4–12

115. Stelling CB, Powell DE, Mattingly SS
Fibroadenomas: histopathology and MR imaging features
Radiology (1987) 162:399–407

116. Stelling CB, Wang PC, Lieber A et al
Prototype coil for magnetic resonance imaging of the female breast
Radiology (1985) 154:457-462

117. Strigl R, Lukas P
Was leistet die Kernspintomographie im Rahmen der Komplementärdiagnostik zur Früherkennung des Mammakarzinoms (Fallberichte)?
in: Alete wissenschaftlicher Dienst (Hrsg)
Proceedings der 20. Tagung der Bayerischen Gesellschaft für Geburtshilfe und Frauenheilkunde 2.–4. 6. 1988, Augsburg
Landshut: Bosch-Druck

118. Szumowski J, Eisen JK, Vinitski S et al
Hybrid methods of chemical shift imaging
J Magn Res Med (1989) 9:379–388

119. Tabar L, Dean PB
The control of breast cancer through mammography screening; what is the evidence?
Radiol Clin North Amer (1987) 25:933–1006

120. Threatt B, Norbeck JM, Ullman NS et al
Thermography and breast cancer: an analysis of a blind reading
Ann NY Acad Sci (1980) 335:501–509

121. Ungeheuer E, Lüders K
Chirurgische Behandlung des Mammakarzinoms
Deut Ärztebl (1978) 4:161

122. Waal JC de, Vaillant W, Baltzer J et al
Erste Erfahrungen mit dem stereotaktischen Diagnosesystem "Mammotest" bei der Diagnostik röntgenologisch unklarer Veränderungen der Brust
Geburtsh Frauenheilk (1985) 45:592–594

123. Weinmann H-J
Eigenschaften von Gd-DTPA und neuer Derivate
in: Bydder GM et al (eds)
Contrast media in MRI
Proceedings of the international workshop
Berlin: Medicom Europe 1990 (in press)

124. Wiener JI, Chako AC, Merten CW et al
Breast and axillary tissue MR imaging: correlation of signal intensities and relaxation times with pathologic findings
Radiology (1986) 160:299–305

125. Wolfram NT, Morgan R, Moran PR et al
Simultaneous MR imaging of both breasts using a dedicated receiver coil
Radiology (1985) 155:241–243

126. Woods JE, Verheyden CN
Pitfalls and problems with subcutaneous mastectomy
Mayo Clin Proc (1980) 55:687–693

127. Zobel BB, Tella S, Confalone D et al
The STIR sequence in the evaluation of breast nodules
Book of Abstracts
Amsterdam: Soc Magn Res in Med (1989) 691

Index